Elements of Pharmacology

Elements of Pharmacology

A primer on drug action

P. J. BENTLEY
*Mount Sinai School of Medicine of
The City University of New York*

CAMBRIDGE UNIVERSITY PRESS

Cambridge
London   New York   New Rochelle
Melbourne   Sydney

Published by the Press Syndicate of the University of Cambridge
The Pitt Building, Trumpington Street, Cambridge CB2 1RP
32 East 57th Street, New York, NY 10022, USA
296 Beaconsfield Parade, Middle Park, Melbourne 3206, Australia

First published 1981

Library of Congress Cataloging in Publication Data
Bentley, P. J.
Elements of pharmacology.
Bibliography: p.
Includes index.
1. Pharmacology. 1. Title. [DNLM: 1. Phar-
macology. QV 4 B477e]
RM300.B456   615′.1   80–26624
ISBN 0 521 23617 7 hard covers
ISBN 0 521 28074 5 paperback

Transferred to digital printing 2003

To Karin

Contents

	Preface	*page*	ix
1	Introduction		1
2	Scope of pharmacology		2
3	Where do drugs come from?		4
4	The names of drugs		7
5	Techniques and methods of pharmacology		10
6	Absorption, distribution, and elimination of drugs; pharmacokinetics		12
7	The nature of responses to drugs		40
8	Receptor theory		44
9	Relationship of chemical structure to biological activity		72
10	Roles of the cell membrane in responses to drugs		79
11	Clinical aspects of the actions of drugs		89
12	Conclusion		138
	References		140
	Glossary of drugs named in the text		145
	Index		153

Preface

This book is the result of a suggestion by an endocrinologist who acted as a referee for a longer concurrent book* that I also wrote. He thought an introductory chapter (my Chapter 2) to that volume might have a more general and wider appeal if presented as an aid to understanding what pharmacology is all about. This origin has contributed to my broad selection of pharmacological examples based on drugs used by endocrinologists. However, receptors for hormones also provide some of the best-studied examples of the drug–receptor concept. Pharmacology impinges on many biological subjects apart from the practice of medicine. The published literature is currently vast, and a plethora of textbooks, usually unavoidably voluminous, is available. This primer is an expanded transcription from the other book, which I hope may provide a small, suitable guide to some fundamentals of pharmacology. It is hoped that it will be useful not only to medical students and practitioners but also to other biologists who may have a general interest in, but limited time to acquaint themselves with this subject.

I would like to thank the referees and editors at Cambridge University Press for encouraging me to write this book. The course in pharmacology given to the medical students at the Mount Sinai School of Medicine provided me with ideas regarding the format. The cooperation of authors and publishers in the production of the illustrations is gratefully acknowledged. My wife, Karin, and graduate student Mary Christine McGahan helped me to organize the material.

P. B.

* *Endocrine pharmacology: physiological basis and therapeutic applications*. Cambridge University Press, Cambridge, Engl., 1980.

1
Introduction

Man is a valetudinary* animal, and is probably unique in this behavior. The availability of drugs† for the treatment of disease offers an opportunity to indulge in this activity. Although it is usually thought that the consequences of taking drugs will be beneficial, or at least pleasurable, the desired effects do not necessarily occur; pills and potions may even be harmful. Iatrogenic or drug-induced diseases are, indeed, becoming quite common. The ultimate effect of a drug will depend primarily on its chemical nature, but it will also be influenced by a variety of other factors, including the quantity used, the state of the person's health, age, sex, diet, heredity, and prior and concurrent use of other types of drugs.

Drugs have undoubtedly provided ways and means for the successful treatment of many human diseases, and the use of drugs for health, pleasure, and profit has increased explosively in the last 30 years. However, drugs are not always used effectively or appropriately, and they are often abused. This situation not only results from their illicit use by those with little or no knowledge of their nature or actions, but it is also the result of an insufficient basic understanding about what may happen to drugs in the body. Although various drugs may behave differently, there is an underlying, common pattern in the behavior of most of them. A knowledge of these principles may provide a rational basis for the therapeutic use of drugs and allow prediction, or at least an understanding, of the responses that may occur. The aim of this primer is to provide a summary of some of the general concepts upon which the subject of *pharmacology,* or the science of drugs, rests.

---

* *Valetudinarian*, one who is constantly concerned about the state of his health.
† *Drug*, an original, simple medicinal substance, organic or inorganic, used by itself or ingested in medicine.

1

2
Scope of pharmacology

The study of the properties of drugs, medicines, and poisons is an old pastime that was originally practiced by the purveyors of medicaments and by professional poisoners. Until the end of the last century drugs were naturally occurring substances, organic or inorganic, most often obtained from plants so that the craft of materia medica (the collection and preparation of such drugs) was closely allied to the science of botany. Large formularies and specifications of such medicines were prepared (pharmacopoeias). The rapid expansion of the chemical industry during the last century has, however, resulted in the introduction of drugs whose numbers far exceed those entered in ancient pharmacopoeias.

Interest in pharmacology has expanded quite amazingly in the twentieth century, and its current growth rate has divided the subject matter into several separate but mutually dependent disciplines. These subdivisions include:

> *Pharmacodynamics*, the effects and mechanisms of actions of drugs on physiological processes.
> *Pharmacotherapeutics* and *clinical pharmacology*, the use of drugs in the treatment of diseases.
> *Toxicology*, the science of poisons. Sometimes considered to be a separate science, toxicology is now often used to include knowledge about the toxic effects of drugs that are used primarily for their therapeutic actions.

Several other specialized areas of pharmacology have now appeared and have received benediction in the form of journals to publish their conclusions. Such disciplines include:

> *Pharmacokinetics*, the quantitative description and prediction of the fate of a drug from the time of its absorption into the body until its biological actions and those of its products are terminated.
> *Pharmacogenetics*, the role of heredity in responses to drugs.
> *Biochemical pharmacology*, the actions of drugs on biochemical processes in the cell.

2

Molecular pharmacology, the description of drug action from a molecular viewpoint. This subject thus includes studies on the relationship of chemical structure to biological activity and on the nature and role of the receptor molecules, by means of which drugs interact with the cell.

Neuropharmacology, the effects of drugs on nerve tissue, especially the brain.

Endocrine pharmacology, the study of hormones as drugs, and of drugs that interact with the endocrine glands and mimic hormonal effects.

Veterinary pharmacology, the specialized use of drugs for the treatment of diseases in animals.

Comparative pharmacology, the study of the effects of drugs on animals but with a view to assessing the general applicability of drug actions, especially with respect to man.

3
Where do drugs come from?

Until the latter part of the nineteenth century, drugs and medicines were all obtained from natural sources, usually plants, sometimes minerals, and occasionally animals. Plants were, however, the predominant sources of drugs, and proliferated considerably as such because of a cultural pooling of herbal remedies, poisons, and pharmaceutical confectionary following the expansion of trade and the geographic explorations in the Middle Ages. In England the leaves of the purple foxglove (*Digitalis purpurea*) provided the cardiac glycosides that are still used to treat congestive heart failure. (The skin of toads was apparently also used as a source of these compounds much earlier in China.) The pain-relieving and pleasurable properties of opium, which is obtained from the seed capsules of the poppy *Papaver somniferum,* were probably first exploited in ancient times in Mesopotamia and Persia. The ubiquitous effects of the *Rauwolfia* alkaloids, which include reserpine, were first utilized in India where they are obtained from the root of the snakeroot plant (*Rauwolfia serpentina*). Today reserpine can be used to control high blood pressure, but it has also enjoyed a vogue in the treatment of psychoses. Tubocurarine is used as a muscle relaxant during anesthesia, but this plant alkaloid (from tropical vines of the family Menispermaceae) was first used as an arrow poison by the Indians who lived around the Amazon river. The bark of the cinchona tree (*Cinchona ledgeriana*), also from South America, is the original source of quinine and quinidine, which are used, respectively, to treat malaria and irregular rhythms of the heartbeat.

Microorganisms have also served as a source of drugs. Ergot, which is obtained from a fungus, *Claviceps purpurea,* that grows on rye, can contract the uterus and has been used to promote labor. Many modern antibiotic drugs also owe their discovery and origins to microorganisms. The most famous example is penicillin, which is produced by *Penicillium* molds. A host of other such antimicrobial chemicals has

4

since been isolated from microorganisms, many of which chemicals are used therapeutically for their selective toxic effects on other types of microorganisms. In some instances they have provided a blueprint for a complete chemical synthesis, whereas others are still made on an industrial scale using microbial cultures. The products made in this way, however, may subsequently be altered by chemical additions so as to improve their usefulness as drugs.

Inorganic, especially metal, compounds have often been used as drugs. Calomel (mercurous chloride) has, for instance, been administered as a laxative, and its diuretic action on the kidneys has, in conjunction with digitalis, been utilized for the treatment of congestive heart failure (in the "Guy's Hospital pill"). These diuretic effects of mercury were independently discovered a second time when an organic mercurial compound (Novasurol) was being tested for its effect in syphilis. This observation led to the introduction of the mercurial diuretic drugs, which, although they have now been superseded, resulted in the development of a contemporary diuretic, ethacrynic acid. Current examples of the use of metal compounds in medicine include gold salts for the treatment of arthritis and platinum compounds for cancer.

The modern organic chemical industry has made two major types of contribution to the provision of drugs. Many naturally occurring substances used as drugs were at first relatively rare and expensive. The ability to chemically synthesize these substances, or related compounds with similar actions, provided considerable medical advances. One of the first such examples was the industrial production of salicylates, substances that can be used to alleviate pain and reduce inflammation and fever. Salicylates were originally extracted from the bark of willow trees, and the chemical synthesis of an even more effective related compound, acetylsalicylic acid (aspirin), made such drugs widely available. The steroid hormones, which are formed by the ovaries, testes, and adrenal cortex, provide another example of the application of chemical techniques to increase the supply of known drugs. These therapeutically useful hormones initially were obtainable only from the glands of animals and from human and animal urine; but these sources of supply are very limited, and such compounds have now been made by steroid chemists. Some of the industrial methods for their preparation, however, include their partial synthesis, with the aid of cultures of microorganisms, using starting materials obtained from plants and bile.

The organic chemical industry has also produced a number of unique original compounds that are used as drugs. The first of these were mainly by-products of the synthetic dye industry. The use of sulfonamide compounds – Prontosil was the first – as antimicrobial drugs was initiated in 1932. One of the side effects of such drugs was observed to be a hypoglycemia, sometimes fatal, which led to the development of the sulfonylurea drugs that are used to lower blood sugar and treat diabetes mellitus. Sulfonamides were also observed to have a weak diuretic effect on the kidney, which provided an important clue resulting in the introduction of the thiazide diuretics. The unique importance of the latter, in contrast to the mercurial diuretics, is that they are effective when taken orally.

A recent technological by-product of molecular biology has been the use of cloned synthetic genes to produce some hormone preparations. Genes for the hormones have been introduced into microorganisms (*Escherichia coli*) that, when so programmed, then produce the hormones. This method has been developed for the commercial production of human insulin and growth hormone and will offer important advances for the treatment of diabetes mellitus and dwarfism due to pituitary disorders in children.

4
The names of drugs

A drug usually has several names. Its *chemical* name, which is in accord with internationally agreed upon rules about naming chemical compounds, provides, to the initiated, a description of its structure. However, this name is often quite long and can also be cumbersome, difficult to remember and to pronounce. Thus most drugs are also provided with a shorter *official*, or *generic*, name, which is easier to remember, and which may receive international recognition under the auspices of the World Health Organization. As no person or company owns it, this is also referred to as the *nonproprietary* name. Some drugs even have popular names, which, in the case of illicit drugs, are often referred to as their "street names" (e.g., methamphetamine = "speed," cocaine = "snow," phenobarbital = "purple hearts").

A pharmaceutical company that markets a drug may have a patent on its production; for this purpose it is usually provided with a *trade*, or *proprietary*, name. This may be shorter than the generic name and is usually intended to be catchier and easier to remember and write. Many drugs are, however, not patented or are made under license by several manufacturers. Thus, a single drug may have many different trade names. As an example: A popular diuretic drug has the generic name chlorothiazide. Its chemical name is 6-chloro-$2H$-1,2,4-benzothiadiazine-7-sulfonamide, 1,1-dioxide. This is an excellent drug that acts orally; tolerance to it does not develop; and it is used widely in the treatment of hypertension and congestive heart failure. It is made by several manufacturers in different countries, who have given it at least 20 trade names, including: Alurene, Chlorosol, Chlorurit, Choltride, Diuresol, Diuril, Diuriliex, Diurite, Exuril, Flumen, Minzil, Neo-dema, Salisan, Saluril, Saluretil, Saluric, Urinex, Warduzide, and Yadulan. This example of a many-named drug is not unique!

There may exist some differences between preparations of a drug

7

even though the main active ingredient is chemically identical in all of them. They may, for instance, be made up in different-sized doses, their physical or crystalline form may vary (polymorphism), or the fillers used to make up bulk in tablets may differ. It has even been claimed that their color may contribute to a placebo effect ("I like the little pink tablets, doctor"). There are also more subtle differences that can occur during the manufacturing process, such as the size of the particles of the drug, the amount of water present in the tablet, and the degree of compression of the material. Such factors may have surprising effects, as they can influence the rate of absorption of the drug. If the tablet does not disintegrate, or if it does so incompletely, much of it will be excreted in the feces. Failure to dissolve satisfactorily may result in a failure to attain therapeutic concentrations in the blood.

In order to try to standardize drug preparations made at different times and in different places, certain chemical, and sometimes biological, criteria have been laid down to which they must conform. Many of these criteria are set out in such handbooks as the *British Pharmacopoeia* (*BP*), the *United States Pharmacopoeia* (*USP*), the *British Pharmaceutical Codex* (*BPC*), and the *United States National Formulary* (*NF*). A disintegration test, which is carried out in a test tube, confirms that a tablet can break up under certain conditions; a dissolution test demonstrates its solubility. Such in vitro tests, however, do not give a perfect prediction of what will happen biologically in the body (in vivo). Unfortunately, a number of differences have been observed in the therapeutic effects of certain preparations of drugs that are chemically equivalent to each other.

One rather dramatic example involves the digitalis cardiac glycoside drug, digoxin. Such drugs are used to increase the force of contraction of cardiac muscle in people suffering from congestive heart failure. Their margin of safety, however, is not great. The differences between therapeutically effective and toxic levels in the plasma can be quite small. Hence it is not surprising that about 25 percent of people who are treated with these drugs develop symptoms of severe intoxication. It was observed that when one brand of digoxin was substituted for another, symptoms of toxicity appeared. Although the two preparations were chemically equivalent, they were not biologically equivalent.

There can be several reasons for such a lack of an equivalent therapeutic effect, including disease and the concurrent use of other drugs. For instance, the thiazide diuretics may produce a hypokalemia, and this lack of electrolyte can increase the effect, and toxicity, of the digitalis drug. It has, however, also been established in several laboratories in different countries that the blood levels of the digoxin may differ substantially following the administration of chemically equivalent doses, but using preparations from different commercial sources (see, e.g., Manninen et al., 1971; Lindenbaum et al., 1971). The differences that were observed in the serum digoxin concentrations were as great as sevenfold, and principally reflected variation in the absorption of the drug from the gut. Such differences not only existed between preparations of digoxin manufactured by various companies, but were also seen between batches made at different times in the same factory. A change in the manufacturing process for digoxin was made by one company, and this change resulted in a doubling of its potency (editorial, 1972). This increase reflected a change in the physical characteristics, and hence the absorption (bioavailability), of the drug. Such problems fortunately are quite rare, but the example does point out difficulties that may occur when a switch is made from one brand, or preparation, of a drug to another. The names of drugs can thus be of practical therapeutic importance.

The names of drugs may also be of financial interest. For a variety of reasons the prices of chemically and, it is hoped, biologically equivalent drugs may vary considerably, sometimes showing several-fold differences. Drugs that go by their generic or nonproprietary names are usually less expensive than their proprietary equivalents. We thus, in our choice of drugs, have the additional problem of a lack of financial equivalence. For the pecunious, or insured, such matters may not be a problem. However, many medical institutions, social welfare services and their supporters, and impecunious individuals must often bear the high costs of drugs. It has therefore often been an expressed wish, or even an official policy and obligation, to request that physicians prescribe, and pharmacists dispense, generic, rather than proprietary, drugs. Such rules have often been highly controversial, and apart from the moral issue of appearing to dictate what a physician or pharmacist may choose to do, involve the ogre of possible differences in biological equivalence or uniformity. It is not so much a question of one drug preparation being "better" than another, but rather that they may not be strictly the same. At present the most practical advice is that the physician should be aware of the groups of drugs in which such problems are likely to occur and where the consequences of a lack of biological equivalence may be serious. Documented instances of such problems have involved, apart from the cardiac glycosides, the anticonvulsant phenytoin, corticosteroids, the oral hypoglycemic tolbutamide, and some anticoagulants and antibiotics.

5
Techniques and methods of pharmacology

Pharmacology, like most other sciences, has the ultimate intention of describing its subject (drugs) in terms of chemistry and physics. It is, however, a biological science and so is concerned with the responses of living systems. For this type of work pharmacology has borrowed techniques from physiology and microbiology but has also developed some methods that are peculiarly its own. Because these procedures utilize changes in the activity of living tissues and cells to make measurements, they are called *bioassays*. The results are expressed in terms of arbitrary *units,* often agreed upon by international committees. These techniques are useful both in research and in the therapeutic application of pharmacology where they are also used for purposes of identification and to confirm purity. Before the era of the chemical preparation of drugs, most medicines were obtained in a relatively impure condition, often as minor components of complex mixtures with other substances. In addition, their chemical nature was usually unknown. Moreover, even when structure is known, chemical analysis is not always feasible. Bioassays may then be useful, and are often essential.

If properly designed almost any type of biological response can be used to give a parameter that can be expressed in quantitative terms. Such methods may involve an intact (in vivo) animal and utilize responses that are as crude as its death, convulsions, or vomiting; or a change in its blood pressure, urine flow, or the levels of metabolites, such as glucose, in the blood. The survival and rates of growth of cultures of microorganisms can also be used for bioassay. Isolated pieces of living organisms, such as a muscle, an endocrine gland, or a slice of an organ, may be kept alive for various periods in culture, ranging from a few hours to many months. These preparations provide in vitro methods for performing bioassays and include such standard laboratory tissues as rat or guinea pig uterus or more exotic preparations like the intestine of a goldfish or the oviduct of a chicken.

The adventurous use of bioassay techniques in research has resulted in the identification of many substances whose existence was unsuspected in nature. These include virtually all of the natural excitants in the body – neurotransmitters and hormones. Many other substances that act as excitants elsewhere, in plants, animals, and microorganisms, were also discovered by such techniques. Recent examples include the prostaglandins and thromboxanes (ubiquitous substances that modulate cell activities), endorphins ("endogenous morphine" – which behave as neuromodulators and whose functions include a blocking of the sensation of pain), and a natural source of vitamin D from a tropical plant, *Solanum malacoxylin*.

The use of many drugs in medicine is still dependent on their standardization using bioassay methods, which are described, for these purposes, in the *United States Pharmacopoeia* and the *British Pharmacopoeia*. They include some hormones, such as insulin and oxytocin (used in labor), virtually all antibiotic drugs, and some vitamins. There are many pharmacologists and clinicians who would like to see biological testing of clinical drugs used more extensively because it might provide more uniformly acting preparations.

Pharmacology uses a vast array of techniques, many of which are purely chemical or physical ones. Histochemical and immunohistochemical procedures have been adopted as an aid in localizing the sites to which drugs go in the body. The methods of the psychologists are used to describe and measure the effects that drugs may have on behavior. Probably the most useful recent advance for facilitating the study of the actions of drugs has been the introduction of radioimmunoassay. This technique provides fast, accurate, and sensitive methods that can be used to measure small quantities of drugs, especially those in the body, and also to investigate what has for a long time been only a pharmacological concept, but is now a reality, the drug receptor.

6

Absorption, distribution, and elimination of drugs; pharmacokinetics

When a drug is administered, it will usually enter the circulation and be rapidly distributed to the remainder of the body fluids and tissues. To be therapeutically effective, it must reach and maintain a certain minimum concentration in the plasma. If, however, a very high level is attained, it may result in toxic effects. The processes involved include the absorption of drugs into the circulation, their transport and distribution to the tissues, and the processes that control their metabolism and elimination from the body. The role of these processes in relation to the final effects of the drug is summarized in Figure 1.

Administration and bioavailability of drugs

Considerations involved in drug administration

The method of administering a drug is dictated by a number of considerations.

Chemical nature of the drug. The chemical nature of drugs is of primary importance. Thus, proteins and polypeptides will be inactivated by the digestive juices and will be ineffective when given by mouth. Absorption across the gastrointestinal mucosa will be favored if the molecules are lipophilic. Despite such absorption, some drugs are still relatively ineffective because when they pass into hepatic-portal circulation and go to the liver, they may be inactivated there. In some cases such as that of the steroidal sex hormones, this process of metabolism can be so effective as to nearly destroy all of the activity before the drug enters the general circulation. Such preparations can, however, often be chemically modified so as to block their metabolism by the liver.

12

A number of drugs, especially hormonal types of preparations, can be absorbed across the mucosa of the mouth, nasal passages, rectum, vagina, and even the bronchial tree. Absorption will be favored in strongly lipophilic compounds, but weaker ones, such as certain peptides, can also be absorbed in this manner. Such routes of administration can be utilized so as to avoid the action of the digestive and hepatic enzymes. For instance, the peptide hormones of the neurohypophysis and hypothalamus can be effectively administered as nasal snuff or nasal spray, antianginal drugs by sublingual buccal administration, the corticosteroid beclomethasone and salbutamol, which are used to treat asthma, by inhalation spray, and prostaglandins by the vaginal route. Such pathways for drug administration have the advantage that injection of the drug is unnecessary, although total absorption is usually difficult to predict. Local inflammatory and allergic reactions at the site of absorption may also occur, especially if the preparation is not pure. This problem occurred with the early preparations of neurohypophysial

Figure 1. A summary of the multiple events and processes that a drug may undergo following its absorption into the body. (From Ariëns, 1966)

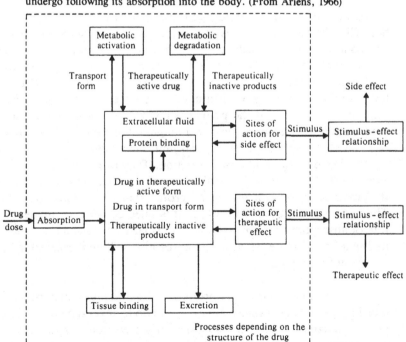

hormones when given as nasal snuff, and also is seen in those who snort cocaine.

Injection or parenteral administration of drugs may be necessary to avoid the digestive tract and to attain and maintain therapeutically effective drug levels in the body. This procedure is especially useful for the polypeptides and proteins, including all the pituitary hormones, insulin, glucagon, and epinephrine. It is also vital for drugs that have an extremely low lipid solubility, such as ganglionic blocking drugs (e.g., hexamethonium). (This property delayed the effective treatment of hypertension.) There are some disadvantages of parenteral administration, the most obvious being the difficulties associated with self-administration (subcutaneous injection is the only really practical method) and the pain and inflammation that may occur at local sites. The latter often reflect the relative impurity of the preparation. Repeated injections at single sites, such as often occur with the use of insulin, can result in local changes, including degeneration of the tissues.

Speed of onset of action. The desired speed of onset of the action of a drug will also influence the choice of a route of administration. Clearly, the intravenous method, such as a single-bolus injection or a continual infusion, will result in the most rapid attainment of therapeutic levels. Such a procedure is usually necessary only in certain crisis situations (e.g., in the rapid and immediate restoration of normal levels of corticosteroids or insulin, or in hypertensive emergencies). In some instances (e.g., if the patient is comatose or vomiting), oral administration will be impractical. Although not as rapid as the intravenous route, the subcutaneous or intramuscular injection of drugs also usually has quite a rapid onset of action. The speed will depend, however, on such factors as the vehicle in which the drug is contained and the presence of contaminants (e.g., proteins) to which it may be bound. The nature of the tissue into which it is injected will also influence its rate of absorption. For instance, it will usually be slowed if it is deposited in adipose tissue, whereas its absorption will be increased if there is a plentiful blood supply.

Duration of action. A prolonged time of action may be desirable. This period may range from a day or two to several months and can be manipulated in several ways. The most common procedure is to modify the physical nature of the drugs, such as by compressing them into pellets or growing large crystals that have a relatively small surface area, or by combining them with vehicles to which they are physically adsorbed or in solution. Chemical combinations, such as the formation of esters, are also used for such purposes.

The steroidal sex hormones can be implanted as pellets, usually subcutaneously, from which they will continue to be absorbed and act for many weeks. Esters of such steroids are also prepared, with periods of action that vary from a few days to 2 or 3 months. It is also possible to control the size of crystalline forms, a characteristic that has been utilized in the preparation of the slowly absorbed (lente) insulins.

To prolong their action, drugs may also be included in special vehicles (e.g., oil) or mixed with proteins where they become enmeshed and adsorbed. Steroid drugs are sometimes prepared and injected in oil. This vehicle has also been used to create slowly absorbable deposits for an ester of antidiuretic hormone (ADH; vasopressin tannate in oil) and for administering iodine in geographic areas (goiter belts) where a deficiency of this element results in thyroid problems. The combination of insulin with proteins such as protamine and globin is used to delay its absorption. Such delayed absorption can create problems because there is a loss in the amount of control, and the vehicles themselves sometimes promote local adverse tissue reactions.

Another method of prolonging the effective absorption of a drug is to create a tissue reservoir by administering it in a form that is rapidly accumulated by a tissue, usually fat, from which it is slowly released. The drug itself may initially be an inactive form, such as the female sex hormone preparation chlorotrianisene, which is metabolized and activated after its release.

Attempts to maintain the levels of drugs and hormone preparations at effective therapeutic, but nontoxic, concentrations has resulted in the development of a number of special mechanical pumps for their delivery. Such devices may be useful for periods of treatment extending over several weeks, such as the chronic administration of anticoagulants, chemotherapeutic drugs in cancer, or antibiotics to combat a difficult infection. Potentially, however, their use could extend to a lifetime, as, for example, for administering insulin to patients with diabetes mellitus. There is evidence that a tight or rigid control of blood glucose levels in such people may help prevent the long-term vascular degeneration that is seen in this disease. There are several types of pump. Small, implantable subcutaneous pumps made from titanium have been tested, which utilize a fluorocarbon vapor–liquid system for producing a pressure to inject a drug. The simplest type of pump used to administer insulin is a portable mechanical device weighing about 300 g, which is attached to a shoulder strap and delivers the hormone to a subcutaneous site on the abdomen (Pickup et al., 1979). The rate is adjustable, and it is speeded up at mealtimes. More sophisticated closed-loop pumps have been developed in which control is exerted via a feedback mechanism, which operates in response to the plasma glucose concentration. This system requires the insertion of a "glucose electrode" into a blood vessel and utilizes a computer to adjust the feedback control. The ultimate practicality of such a system is not, however, clear at this time.

Local administration. Localized administration of drug preparations is often used to treat a lesion directly, and may afford the most convenient method of attaining and maintaining high therapeutically effective concentrations. Such a procedure may indeed be essential to avoid general systemic concentrations of drugs that may have unacceptable side effects. Corticosteroids are used in this way to exert an antiinflammatory action by direct topical application on the skin and cornea, injection intraarticularly into joints, insertion into the rectum, and inhalation into the bronchi. Catecholamines are administered by inhalation to dilate the bronchi. Many ophthalmic drugs are applied topically, including some (e.g., pilocarpine) that are used to treat glaucoma. Problems may sometimes occur owing to the absorption of the drug from such sites into the general circulation. Such effects may, however, be relatively localized, as may be seen in a degeneration of underlying cutaneous tissues or increases in intraocular pressure that are sometimes associated with prolonged topical uses of corticosteroids. The use of corticosteroids to treat asthma has also resulted in problems due to systemic absorption, which occurs even when they are applied directly in the form of inhalation sprays. Chemical analogues have been developed that exhibit high local activity but are not appreciably absorbed. Vasoconstrictor drugs (e.g., epinephrine) are sometimes added to preparations such as local anesthetics that are injected into sites where localized action is required.

Bioavailability

Although successful intravenous administration of a drug assures absorption, the process is not necessarily completed when other routes are used. The proportion, or fraction, of a drug that is absorbed into the circulation following its administration is called its bioavailability (see Koch-Weser, 1974a,b). The problem of partial absorption of a drug is perhaps most obvious when one is considering its oral administration, but absorption may also be incomplete, because of local inactivation or binding, when the drug is given intramuscularly or subcutaneously.

Some of the many factors that can influence a drug's bioavailability after oral administration are shown in Table 1. They include conditions

Table 1. *Factors influencing bioavailability and absorption of drugs from the gastrointestinal tract*

Factors affecting bioavailability of orally administered drugs
1. Drug characteristics
     Inactivation before gastrointestinal absorption
     Incomplete absorption
     Biotransformation in intestinal wall or liver
2. Formulation of drug product
     State of the drug
     Excipients
3. Interaction with other substances in the gastrointestinal tract
     Food
     Drugs
4. Patient characteristics
     Gastrointestinal pH
     Gastrointestinal motility
     Gastrointestinal perfusion
     Gastrointestinal flora
     Gastrointestinal structure
     Malabsorption states
     Hepatic function
     Genetic makeup

Drug interactions in the gut that can influence absorption of drugs
1. Change in gastric or intestinal pH (antacids)
2. Change in gastrointestinal motility (cathartics, motility depressants)
3. Change in gastrointestinal perfusion (cardiovascular drugs)
4. Interference with mucosal function (neomycin, colchicine)
5. Chelation (tetracycline with calcium or magnesium)
6. Exchange resin binding (cholestyramine with acidic drugs)
7. Adsorption (charcoal, kaolin, antacids)
8. Solution in poorly absorbable liquid (mineral oil)
9. Unknown mechanisms (heptabarbital with bishydroxycoumarin; phenobarbital with griseofulvin; allopurinol with warfarin)

Source: Koch-Weser (1974a). Adapted by permission from *The New England Journal of Medicine 291:* 235.

in the gastrointestinal tract such as the pH, motility, the actions of microorganisms that may metabolize the drug, the temporal relationship to meals, and the presence of other drugs.

Different species of drugs obviously may exhibit different characteristics with respect to the degree of completeness of their absorption from a particular site. In addition, there has been an increasing number of reports of variations in bioavailability among proprietary brands and formulations of the same generic drug (see Chapter 4). In some instances, differences between preparations of a drug can be related to the time required for it to disintegrate and dissolve (*dissolution time*) in vitro.

Differences in bioavailability that are not readily predictable can lead to clinical problems (see Chapter 4), such as the administration of ineffective doses or unexpected toxicities. These problems can arise when one is simply changing from one brand of a drug to another.

Distribution and binding of drugs

Dispersal of drugs

When a drug enters the circulation, either following absorption from the gut or by injection, it is rapidly diluted and dispersed, so that its local concentration declines rapidly. It does not, however, necessarily enter all the fluid compartments or tissues with equal facility, if at all. This process of distribution is an important practical consideration because a drug may, for instance, have difficulty in maintaining an effective concentration or in reaching sites where its therapeutic effect may be desired. Conversely, it may gain access to undesirable places, where it may exert toxic or side effects.

There are several barriers that can restrict the movement of drugs in the body, notably, the capillaries, which limit movement into the interstitial fluids; the blood–brain barrier, which controls access to the brain; and the cell membrane. There are also barriers inside the cell, and the ability of drugs to enter the mitochondria or the lipid vesicles of the endoplasmic reticulum can influence their metabolism. Generally, access across such membranes is promoted if the drugs are lipid-soluble; water-soluble molecules, especially large ones and those that are ionized, gain access with more difficulty. Binding to the tissues, especially to plasma proteins, will also limit dispersal, as will ready solubility in the fat stores of adipose tissue.

Drug binding to and displacement from plasma proteins

Many drugs bind to plasma proteins (see Koch-Weser and Sellers, 1976a,b). In many instances where this occurs, less than 5 percent of the total drug in the plasma is in its "free," unbound state. The albumins are the most plentiful of the plasma proteins and provide the largest number of potential binding sites, but other plasma proteins, especially the globulins, are often more specific with respect to the substances with which they react. They therefore have only a low capacity to bind a drug or hormone, but they do so quite strongly (they have a high affinity). Binding to plasma proteins is usually a reversible process (covalent binding occurs only rarely), and there is an equilibrium between the bound drug and that which is free in solution. The number of binding sites on a protein is limited, so that it is saturable. The binding of two or more substances may thus be interfered with because of competition among the substances for the same sites, or the occupation of adjacent positions so that the substances interfere with each other. Drugs often share such binding sites; so they can displace each other.

The mutual displacement of drugs from binding sites on plasma proteins can have dramatic effects on their actions in the body. These effects are related not only to changes in levels of the free form of the drug, which is the biologically active form, but they can also alter the rate of elimination of the compound from the body. Initially, however, one may expect an exaggerated and even toxic effect when one drug displaces another from a binding site. Because the active free fraction of the drug may represent only 1 or 2 percent of the total amount in the blood, a quite modest displacement from the predominant remaining proportion attached to plasma proteins can have a large effect on the unbound drug. Such a change can be of considerable importance clinically; for instance, it may result in hemorrhage in patients being treated with anticoagulants such as warfarin, or in hypoglycemia in diabetic patients who are taking tolbutamide. Both of these drugs are bound to plasma proteins, and they may mutually displace each other. Such an event may occur in the presence of several types of drugs (Table 2).

Other changes occur subsequent to the displacement of drug and may mask or modify the change. These responses are the result of attainment of a new steady state as a result of redistribution of the drug and changes in the rate of its elimination. The expected changes in serum concentration and the processes concerned with elimination of the drug are summarized in Table 3. When the amount of unbound drug in the serum is increased, the drug will be free to move into other fluid compartments; a decrease in concentration results from this redistribution. Filtration of the drug across the glomerulus will also be enhanced,

Table 2. *Clinically important interactions between drugs that result in their displacement from binding to plasma proteins*

Displaced drug	Displacing drug	Possible clinical consequences
Warfarin and other highly albumin-bound coumarins (anti-coagulants)	Clofibrate Ethacrynic acid Mefenamic acid Nalidixic acid Oxyphenbutazone Phenylbutazone Trichloroacetic acid (metabolite of chloral hydrate)	Excessive hypopro-thrombinemia; hemorrhage
Tolbutamide (oral hypoglycemic drug)	Phenylbutazone Sulfaphenazole Salicylates	Hypoglycemia

Source: Koch-Weser and Sellers (1976b). Adapted by permission from *The New England Journal of Medicine* 294:527.

Table 3. *Consequences of displacement of drug from binding to serum albumin*

	Immediately after displacement	New steady state
Free drug fraction in serum	Increased	Increased
Free drug concentration in serum	Increased	Unchanged
Total drug concentration in serum	Unchanged	Decreased
Pharmacologic activity	Increased	Unchanged
Glomerular filtration	Increased	Unchanged
Tubular secretion	Variable	Unchanged
Diffusion into liver cell	Increased	Unchanged
Active hepatic uptake	Variable	Unchanged

Source: Koch-Weser and Sellers (1976b). Adapted by permission from *The New England Journal of Medicine* 294:528.

so that drug excretion via the urine will be increased. The effects on renal tubular secretion of a drug are variable, but if active transport is involved in this process, the secretion rate will be unchanged, or decreased. The reason is that the rate of dissociation of a drug from plasma proteins is so fast that binding will not normally limit the rate of active transport. Thus, no significant change in serum levels of the drug will be expected. However, if, as a result of redistribution, the total concentration of the drug in the serum declines, active transport-mediated excretion will decline. The same arguments apply to an active transport process that may be involved in the drug's access to other sites, especially the liver. Diffusion to metabolic sites in the liver will, however, be increased as a result of displacement from plasma proteins so that the drug's metabolism will be enhanced. Thus, a new steady-state equilibrium will be attained in which the total drug in the serum will be decreased, but the free, biologically active portion will be similar to its initial value. This does not mean that dosages of drugs need not be adjusted in the expectation of mutual displacement of drugs from plasma-protein binding; indeed, it is only by doing this that one can avoid possible *acute* toxic responses.

Concentrations of specific binding proteins

The concentrations of specific binding proteins in plasma exhibit some lability, which is related to the physiological circumstances and may be altered in response to disease and therapy. Increases in plasma proteins, which can bind the increased steroid hormones, occur in pregnancy. The therapeutic administration of estrogens may have similar effects. Plasma protein concentrations, including those of the albumins, may decrease in certain conditions, especially in the presence of liver and renal disease. Changes in the particular protein composition of the plasma may also have qualitative effects that decrease the binding of drugs. As the unbound concentrations of many drugs are relatively small compared to the bound fraction, quite modest declines in binding can have large effects on the free therapeutically active concentrations of a drug. It may thus be necessary to adjust the dosage of drugs in such diseases in order to maintain their therapeutic action or avoid toxic side effects. However, changes in elimination will often be sufficient to compensate for such effects, especially as changes in plasma protein concentrations are usually gradual and quite slow in their onset.

Metabolism, or biotransformation, of drugs

The chemical structures of drugs can be altered as a result of enzymically controlled metabolic activities at various sites in the body. Such modifications in molecular structure change various properties of the molecule, including its biological activity and solubility. These changes usually result in a reduction or abolition of its actions (inactivation) and an increase in its water solubility, which facilitates its excretion in the urine and bile. There are, however, a number of occasions when the effectiveness of drugs is enhanced as a result of their metabolism so that an activation is said to occur. In other instances, metabolites may retain an appreciable amount of the original activity, or they may have other effects, including toxic actions.

The metabolism of drugs may occur in any tissue in the body. Some of the enzymes involved (e.g., peptidases and esterases) often have quite nonspecific effects with respect to particular drugs and have a ubiquitous distribution. In other instances, however, special enzymes are found predominantly in certain tissues. The liver plays a central and predominant role in the metabolism of most drugs, but the kidney and gastrointestinal tract are also important, and in certain instances tissues as diverse as the brain, lungs, prostate, placenta, and the blood plasma may be involved. The target, or effector, tissues can be sites for drug metabolism. Metabolism of drugs may occur at either extracellular or intracellular sites. The latter are especially important and are associated with various cellular structures, including the smooth endoplasmic reticulum (SER, in the microsomal fraction), mitochondria, and the "cell sap" (the supernatant fraction).

Drugs can be enzymically assaulted in a host of ways. Most compounds, however, are predominantly metabolized in a quite specific manner, which is dictated by their chemical structure and the sites where they tend to accumulate in the body. In some instances, this may involve the action of a single enzyme, but usually there is a chain of reactions which result in the progressive availability of substrates that are formed stepwise from the biotransformations of the drugs. Thus, a side chain may be progressively attacked and shortened, or a hydroxyl group may be formed that provides a site for the combination of the drug with such moieties as sugars, amino acids, and sulfuric acid. The types of metabolic changes in drugs can be divided into two main groups:

1. *Nonsynthetic* or *degradative reactions*, which involve such processes as oxidation, reduction, and hydrolysis, and include deamination, dealkylation, dehalogenation, and hydroxylation.
2. *Synthetic* or *conjugation reactions*, which involve the attachment of new components, such as glucuronide, sulfate, glycine, acetate, and methylation.

Because synthetic reactions usually succeed nonsynthetic ones, the two types have also been referred to as phase I and II reactions.

Extracellular metabolism of drugs

Extracellular metabolism of drugs occurs in the digestive fluids, the plasma, and the interstitial fluids in the proximity or possibly at the surface of cells. Such processes would be expected to be relatively more important for substances that have difficulty in entering cells, especially large water-soluble molecules and those for which no specific mechanism for cellular uptake exists. Thus, many peptides are attacked by trypsin and chymotrypsin-like enzymes, carboxypeptidases, and aminopeptidases, which are extruded by cells and may be activated in the extracellular fluids. Such processes, however, also undoubtedly occur inside cells.

Esterases are plentiful in the extracellular fluids of the gastrointestinal tract, as a result of both the actions of the digestive enzymes and the activities of bacteria. The latter are of special interest with respect to their actions in hydrolyzing conjugated compounds, notably glucuronides that are secreted in the bile. Esterases, such as cholinesterase, are responsible for metabolizing such drugs as succinylcholine, aspirin, and several local anesthetics.

Intracellular metabolism of drugs

Intracellular metabolism of drugs, which is of predominant importance, depends of course on the drugs' ability to enter the cell. Lipid solubility or a specific uptake process, or pump, will favor these processes. Biotransformation may be due to soluble enzymes in the cytoplasm, or it may take place in the mitochondria or as a result of reactions that occur with the components of the smooth endoplasmic reticulum. The activity of the latter structure is particularly important in the liver. Compounds must be lipid-soluble in order to gain access to the drug-metabolizing components of the endoplasmic reticulum.

Metabolism by cytoplasmic enzymes. The cytoplasm contains many soluble enzymes, among them methyltransferases, which add methyl groups to drugs and hormones. One of the best known is catechol-*O*-methyltransferase (COMT; scheme 1) which plays an im-

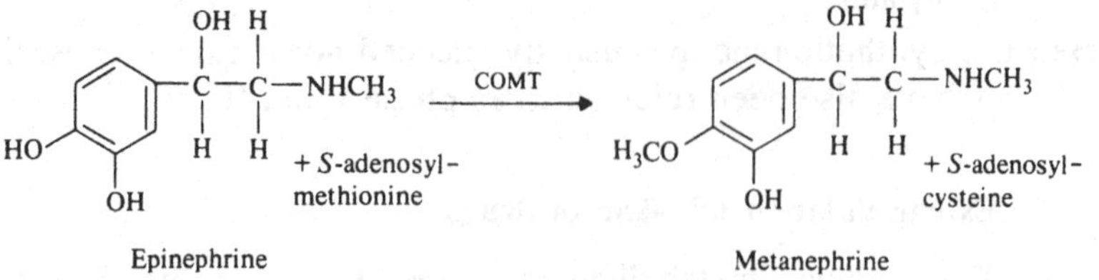

Scheme 1

portant role in the inactivation of catecholamines such as epinephrine. These methylation reactions involved the utilization of the cofactor *S*-adenosylmethionine, which is formed from ATP and methionine. N- and S-methylation also occur. (Methyltransferases are also present in the microsomes.)

Sulfokinase (or sulfotransferase) enzymes have also been identified in the cytoplasm. These enzymes promote the synthesis of sulfate conjugates or esters of drugs, including steroidal drugs, morphine, and phenobarbital. The reaction involves an intermediate, 3'-phospho-adenosine-5'-phosphosulfate, known as "active sulfate" or PAPS, formed from SO_4^{2-} and ATP (scheme 2). Sulfation can occur at either the O or NH positions.

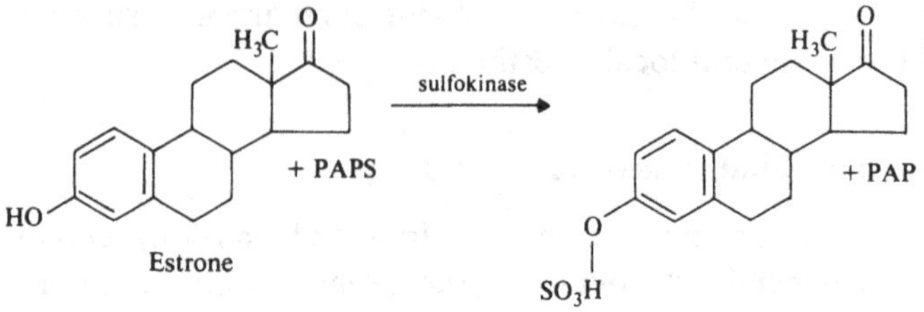

Scheme 2

Metabolism by mitochondrial enzymes. The mitochondria are the site of a number of oxidizing enzymes, including monoamine oxidase (MAO), which acts on some amines, such as epinephrine and 5-hydroxytryptamine (scheme 3). Monoamine oxidase is an important site of action for a group of antidepressant drugs; their inhibition of this enzyme can result in many side effects in the body.

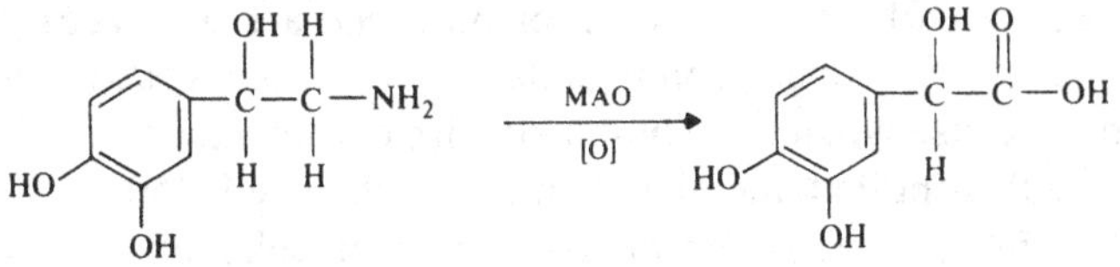

Norepinephrine   2,4-Dihydroxymandelic acid

Scheme 3

Acetylation is an important type of conjugation reaction which is associated with mitochondrial function and is responsible for the biotransformation of a number of drugs, such as hydralazine, isoniazid, phenelzine, and sulfonamides. It occurs in the liver. Acetic acid can become conjugated to drugs via its "activation" by CoA to form acetyl-CoA. The acyl group can then be transferred onto an amino group of a drug (scheme 4). Some individuals have a poor ability to

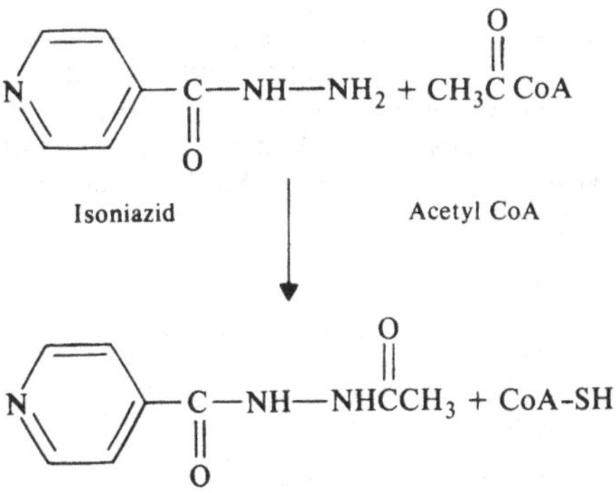

Isoniazid   Acetyl CoA

Acetylisoniazid

Scheme 4

metabolize drugs via this reaction because of a deficiency that has a genetic basis (see Chapter 11, under "Genetic differences in drug responses") and can influence the therapeutic use of such drugs.

Metabolism by oxidation reactions. The microsomal system that oxidizes many drugs is unique as it utilizes a reverse transport of electrons that reduces or "activates" molecular oxygen. This process has been best characterized in the liver, but all the details are not yet understood, and some are arguable and may differ from tissue to tissue. There are several components of this mixed oxidase system (as two substrates, NADPH, and the drug or hormone are oxidized), but the central one is a heme-iron protein called *cytochrome P-450*. It was given this name because when it is combined with carbon monoxide, it exhibits a strong absorption band at 450 nm. Cytochrome P-450 can combine with many drugs, steroid hormones, and molecular oxygen, the last being reduced and incorporated into the drug. The entire cycle of events is called the *cytochrome P-450 oxygenase system*.

The electrons, or reducing equivalents, are derived as a result of the oxidation of reduced nicotinamide adenine dinucleotide phosphate, NADPH (or possibly also NADH). The sequence of events is shown in Figure 2. The drug (or steroid) combines with the oxidized form of the cytochrome P-450, which is reduced. This process involves the enzyme *NADPH–cytochrome c reductase*, which appears to be identical to what was formerly called NADPH–cytochrome P-450 reductase. It is thought that a microsomal *non-heme-iron protein*, which carries the

Figure 2. Cytochrome P-450 oxygenase cycle. The electrons (or reducing equivalents) are derived from the oxidation of NADPH to NADP$^+$. The reduced non-heme-iron protein (NH-Fe^{2+} protein) is a microsomal constituent that *may be* an intermediary in this transfer from NADPH to cytochrome P-450. Further electrons are also derived from NADPH and are thought to be transferred from cytochrome b_5.

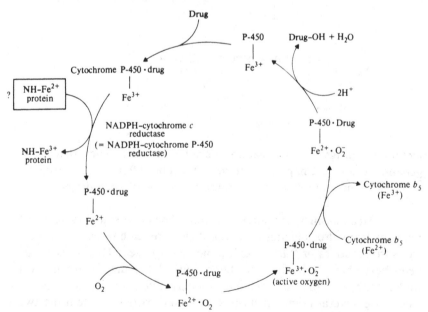

electrons to the cytochrome P-450, is involved as an intermediary in this reaction. The reduced cytochrome P-450 drug complex then combines with molecular O_2 which is then said to be "activated." Additional electrons are passed from the NADPH or NADH system via cytochrome b_5 and upon the acquisition of 2H the complex dissociates into the oxidized drug, H_2O, and oxidized cytochrome P-450. This microsomal system usually mediates hydroxylation reactions, but oxidation at other sites, including C, N, and S, is possible, so that deamination, desulfuration, and dealkylation reactions occur. Examples of drugs that are oxidized in this manner include phenytoin, meperidine, quinine, morphine, and chlorpromazine. Exogenous "pollutants" including insecticides and carcinogenic chemicals may also be metabolized in this way. Cytochrome P-450–mediated reactions also occur, but to a lesser extent, in other tissues, including adrenalcortical mitochondria, the placenta, the kidney, and the gastrointestinal tract. Several other types of cytochrome P-450 have been identified with different absorption bands. There thus appears to be a family of such proteins that may each be preferentially involved in the metabolism of certain types of drugs.

Glucuronide conjugation also occurs in the liver microsomes and involves the formation of activated glucuronic acid or uridine diphosphate glucuronic acid from glucose-1-phosphate and uridine triphosphate, UTP, in a series of enzymic reactions. The final reaction, which occurs in the microsomes, is:

$$\text{UDP–glucuronic acid} + \text{ROH} \xrightarrow[\text{transferase}]{\text{glucuronyl}} \text{RO–glucuronide} + \text{UDP}$$

Many drugs, including those that are phenols, carboxylic acids, and aromatic amines, are conjugated with glucuronide, among them the salicylates, morphine, chloramphenicol, and steroidal drugs, such as the sex hormones. Such metabolites appear in the urine and bile. This type of conjugation also occurs at other sites on molecules, such as NH, S, and ester groups.

Metabolism by reduction reactions. The metabolism of drugs by reduction reactions is not common but can be important, especially for steroids. Saturation of double bonds and carbonyl groups in such compounds is an important process in their metabolism, including inactivation and activation. These types of reactions may involved NADH or

NADPH as an H donor. The precise location of the enzymes in the cells is not always clear, but microsomal, nonmicrosomal, and nuclear sites have been identified. Two examples of such reactions are shown in schemes 5 and 6. In scheme 5, the hypnotic drug chloral hydrate is

$$\underset{\text{Chloral hydrate}}{Cl_3C - CHO.H_2O} \xrightarrow[\text{alcohol dehydrogenase}]{\text{NADH}} \underset{\text{Trichloroethanol}}{Cl_3 - CH_2OH} + H_2O$$

Scheme 5

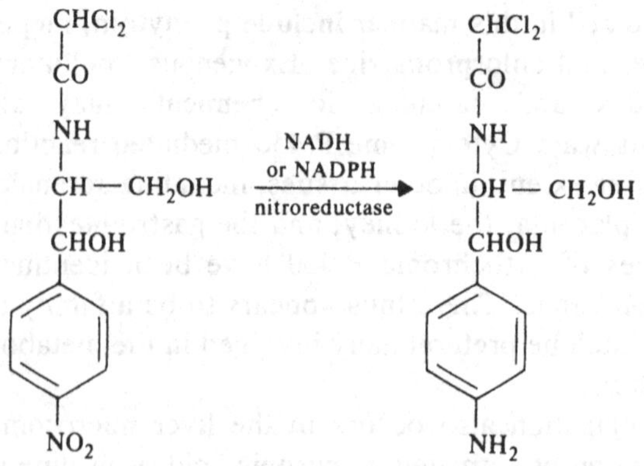

Chloramphenicol Aminochloramphenicol

Scheme 6

converted to its active metabolite trichloroethanol by *nonmicrosomal enzymes*. In scheme 6, *microsomal enzymes* mediate a nitro reduction of the antibiotic chloramphenicol.

Dehalogenation can involve reduction, if the halogen is replaced by a hydrogen, or oxidation, as in the removal of a hydrogen (dehydrohalogenation). Such a reaction is involved in the metabolism of halogen-containing anesthetics such as halothane, and toxic chemicals such as carbon tetrachloride and DDT. A deiodinase enzyme has a ubiquitous distribution in the body, where it is concerned with the transformation of the tetraiodo compound thyroxine (T_4) to the more active triiodothyronine (T_3).

Factors influencing drug metabolism

The rate of metabolism, and clearance, of drugs can vary considerably; in man, a sixfold range is thought to be normal. Such differences appear to reflect nutritional, environmental, and genetic factors. There may also be sexual differences. It should be emphasized that interspecific differences exist (see Chapter 11, under "Genetic differences in drug responses") so that one must be careful in extrapolating results gained from animal experiments. Considerable variation can occur in man, which is related to disease and prior exposure to drugs and environmental contaminants. Newborn infants have a very poor capacity to metabolize drugs, but this ability develops rapidly in the first year of life. Such differences in the ability to metabolize drugs and eliminate them from the body can have important consequences with respect to their therapeutic actions and possible side effects. One of the most obvious situations in which possible changes in the elimination of a drug must be considered is in liver and kidney disease, when there often may be a dramatic decline in this process. The use of drugs in infants also needs considerable circumspection. In these days of polypharmacy, when several drugs are often administered concurrently, interactions (see Chapter 11, under "Drug interactions") that may involve changes in their metabolism are an increasing problem.

Several factors can influence the rate of drug metabolism by tissues, but two are predominant: their blood supply and their innate metabolic ability to carry out biotransformational changes. The binding of drugs to plasma proteins and their tissue storage, such as in adipose tissue, also affect drug metabolism. In advanced liver disease, such as cirrhosis, all these factors may be involved: a decreased blood supply, an inhibition of tissue metabolic activity, and a decline in plasma proteins. Pregnancy can also alter drug metabolism because of changes in the production of binding proteins in plasma, and the additional activity of the placenta and the fetal liver.

The drug-metabolizing activity of the smooth endoplasmic reticulum may be altered in a number of ways. First, as these reactions are usually saturable, and exhibit an exponential course, competition between drugs for metabolism can occur. Because of the very large capacity of such enzymic processes for these substrates, this form of inhibition is, however, rarely seen except under in vitro conditions. Attempts have been made to synthesize inhibitors of the enzymes concerned, and such an experimental drug is SKF 525A (β-diethylaminoethyl-2,2-diphenylpentanoate). Such compounds may bind to essential sites, including cytochrome P-450, in a competitive or noncompetitive manner. Because such enzyme reactions have a widespread physiological role, it is not surprising to find that such drugs are of doubtful therapeutic use. A sufficient degree of selectivity to influence a drug's metabolism without upsetting normal physiological processes may not be possible.

Second, the enzymes and associated proteins and lipids of the smooth endoplasmic reticulum can increase in response to certain stimuli, including many drugs. This *induction* of the microsomal enzyme system appears to be most important in the liver. More than 200 drugs and toxic compounds have been shown to elicit this response; they include a range of drug types, among them some hypnotics, sedatives, anesthetics, and steroids. (See Table 4.) A number of polycyclic hydrocarbon compounds, which are present in tobacco smoke and insecticides (e.g., DDT and dieldrin), also can induce hepatic microsomal enzymes. The prototype of such compounds is the barbiturate phenobarbital. After several days' administration of this hypnotic drug, there is an increase in the size of the liver, and a large proliferation of the smooth endoplasmic reticulum. These changes are associated with an increase in many liver enzymes, but especially the microsomal ones associated with the cytochrome P-450 oxygenase system. The change reflects a de novo protein synthesis and can be inhibited by actinomycin D or puromycin. The response appears to be elicited by the binding of the drug to the cytochrome P-450. However, the drug does not need to be metabolized in order to initiate the response. The effect is relatively nonspecific, as the metabolism of a variety of other drugs is also made possible by the additional microsomal enzymes (an increase that is usually about twofold in man). There are, however, instances when the effect may be relatively specific, such as with 3,4-benzpyrene, which induces enzymes that will metabolize the analgesic acetanilid but not the anesthetic hexobarbital. Drugs that induce microsomal enzymes must be lipid-soluble and preferably should have a relatively prolonged period of action.

The structure of drugs can be modified in order to change the rate of their metabolism and excretion and so alter the time of their action in the body. Thus, substitution of certain amino acids or the removal of terminal amino groups can limit the abilities of enzymes to attack peptide chains so that they are protected and their effects are prolonged. Substitution of a halogen, a Cl for a methyl group, results in a decreased metabolism of the oral hypoglycemic drug chlorpropamide as compared to tolbutamide. The ability of enzymes to change the structure of certain drugs and so activate them may also be utilized to prolong their action, as is seen in the preparation of peptides with additional, protective, terminal chains of amino acids, and in the esterification of steroids. Such compounds can often persist in inactive form for relatively long periods of time in the body, but as a result of their metabolism, they are slowly changed to their active form.

Table 4. *Some drugs that can induce formation of microsomal enzymes, especially in the liver, and thus enhance rates of their own metabolism and that of other drugs*

Hypnotics, sedatives, and anticonvulsants
Phenobarbital and other barbiturates
Glutethimide
Ethanol[a]
Chloral hydrate[a]
Phenytoin
Primidone
Tranquilizers and antipsychotic drugs
Chlorpromazine
Meprobamate
Chlordiazepoxide
Imipramine
Antiinflammatory drugs
Phenylbutazone
Aminopyrine
Corticosteroids
Sulfonamides
Tolbutamide
Carbutamide
Sulfaphenazone
Steroids
Androgens
Estradiol[a]
Corticosteroids
Vitamin D_2 and D_3
Assorted drugs
Mitotane (*o,p'*-DDD)[a]
Metyrapone[a]
Bishydroxycoumarin
Insecticides (e.g., DDT, dieldrin)
Polycyclic hydrocarbons (e.g., cigarette smoke)

[a] First depress then stimulate.

Excretion of drugs

Drugs and their metabolites can be excreted through several pathways. The most important of these is the urine, followed by the bile, but the other gastrointestinal secretions, the sweat, and even the milk of lactating women can also contribute to excretion. The lungs may be important in certain instances, involving substances that are readily vaporized, such as many general anesthetics. Compounds that are completely dependent on such channels for their elimination from the body usually have a relatively long half-life compared to those drugs that undergo metabolism in the body.

The secretion of urine by the kidneys involves filtration of the plasma across the glomerulus, followed, in the renal tubule, by an assortment of processes of reabsorption from the filtrate back into the blood and secretion of solutes by the renal tubular cells into the urine. Apart from ultrafiltration at the glomerulus, these processes involve diffusion and active transport. The filtration of a substance will depend on its size, which will influence its ability to pass across the glomerulus. Drugs bound to plasma proteins thus will not be readily filtered. The lipid solubility of the compound will have an important effect on its ability to diffuse back into the blood, so that hydrophilic molecules and those salts that exist in a dissociated, electrically charged form will tend to be retained in the urine. The excretion of lipid-soluble drugs will, however, be very slow; and for excretion to occur they must be metabolized to more water-soluble forms. Some water-soluble solutes may, however, be reabsorbed from the glomerular filtrate via aqueous channels and by processes involving active transport. Secretion of a number of compounds can occur across the renal tubule, involving the water-soluble ionic forms of certain acids and bases. These secretion "pumps" are dependent on metabolic activity, they are saturable, and their actions can be inhibited competitively by related compounds. Renal diseases clearly may influence the urinary excretion of a drug from the body and necessitate reconsideration of its dose or even its use.

Some drugs, following their metabolic processing in the liver, are excreted in water-soluble form in the bile and thus pass into the intestine. Such compounds, which include a number of steroids, are usually in hydrophilic form, owing largely to their conjugation to glucuronide and sulfate. These conjugated compounds are not readily absorbed from the gut, and if unchanged will be excreted in the feces. However, they may be altered by tissue and bacterial enzymes in the digestive tract and reassume their lipophilic characteristics so that they can be reabsorbed into the circulation. Their elimination will thus be delayed as a result of their being trapped in this cycle of enterohepatic circulation. The prolonged action of the laxative phenolphthalein is due to this effect. Small quantities of such drugs will, however, inevitably "escape" and be excreted in either the feces or the urine.

A number of drugs and their metabolic products, some of which retain biological activity, are excreted in the urine. A well-known example is penicillin. When supplies of this antibiotic were scarce during World War II, the urine of patients was reprocessed to recover the drug. The conjugated estrogen hormones and gonadotropins are excreted in the urine and provide an important source of such substances for therapeutic use.

Drugs can sometimes be excreted in the milk, and the mammary tissue itself may contribute to their metabolism, so that lactation can influence their clearance from the circulation. It can, of course, also provide an undesirable source of drugs for the infant. Some laxatives may be accumulated by infants in this manner.

Pharmacokinetics

The general principles that can be used to describe and predict the behavior of the levels of drugs in the body are called *pharmacokinetics*. Pharmacokinetic analysis facilitates the temporal description, in mathematical terms, of the effects of absorption, distribution, metabolism, and excretion on the levels of a drug in the body (see Greenblatt and Koch-Weser, 1975a,b). Such studies are useful because they may provide data and methods by which the clinician can predict such important parameters as the dosage of a drug that is necessary to attain a given therapeutic concentration and the frequency at which the drug must be administered to maintain such levels.

Certain assumptions are made, and different models can be applied for such mathematical analyses of changing drug levels in the body. The particular ones used are undoubtedly simpler than the actual situation that exists in the body, but they can nevertheless provide useful information. The simplest model (Figure 3a) assumes that the drug is present in a one-compartment system into which drugs can be ab-

34   *Elements of pharmacology*

sorbed, and from which they can be irreversibly eliminated as a result of metabolism and excretion (k_a and k_e are the absorption and elimination rate constants, respectively).

A slightly more complex model (Figure 3b), which approaches the in vivo situation more closely, is the two-compartment system. The central compartment (1) can be considered as being synonymous with the plasma and interstitial fluids of highly perfused organs, such as the liver, kidney, and heart. The contents of this compartment are in equilibrium with the peripheral compartment (2), which corresponds to the tissues and the interstitial fluids in less well-perfused organs. The rate constants for the movements of drug between these two compartments are called k_{12} and k_{21}. Absorption of the dose of the drug and its irreversible elimination are both considered to take place in the central compartment.

For mathematical treatment the rates of the exchanges are considered to be directly proportional to the concentration of the drug (first-order kinetics). However, some drugs do not behave in this way, such as when their elimination may involve facilitated diffusion or active

Figure 3. Schematic models that can be used to describe the distribution and pharmacokinetic behavior of drugs. (a) One-compartment "open" model. (b) Two-compartment "open" model. k_a, absorption rate constant; C, drug concentration; V_d, apparent volume of drug distribution; k_e, elimination rate constant; k_{12} and k_{21}, rate constants for movements of drugs between compartments 1 and 2. First-order (i.e., concentration-dependent) kinetics are considered to apply to k_a, k_e, and k_{12} and k_{21}.

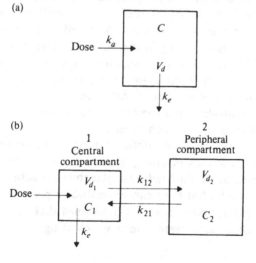

transport, so that saturation may occur (at saturation zero-order kinetics is followed).

The basic information that is required to make mathematical predictions of pharmacokinetic parameters is the administered dose (D or D_0) and subsequent serial measurements of changes in serum concentration of the drug. Such serum values, following oral administration of a drug, can be plotted graphically as shown in Figure 4. The drug levels can be seen to show an initial, relatively fast rise; a peak concentration; and finally a slower decline. A slightly more detailed analysis following intravenous administration of a drug is shown in Figure 4b. In this instance, the drug concentration in the serum rises more rapidly and, after reaching a maximum, declines rapidly. This initial fast decrease reflects the redistribution of the drug between the central compartment and the peripheral compartment and has been called *phase alpha,* with a slope (units of minutes^{-1}) called α. Subsequently, there is an abrupt change in this slope and a slower decline ensues. This is called *phase beta* and reflects the irreversible elimination of the drug as a result of its excretion and metabolism (its slope is called β). This is the elimination rate constant k_e (which is in units of minutes^{-1}).

Using such mathematical and graphical data, one can calculate (Table 5) such values as the total apparent volume of distribution (V_d), the elimination rate constant (k_e), the half-life ($t_{1/2}$), and the clearance rate. This information can be useful clinically, as in the calculation of dosage and the schedule for administration, so as to assure therapeutic, but nontoxic, drug levels in the body. Multiple doses of a drug are often necessary to maintain effective therapeutic levels in the blood, so that correct spacing of the doses is important. If a drug is given too frequently, accumulation can occur, and toxic levels are thus attained; but, conversely, if the drug is given at long intervals, therapeutic levels may not be maintained. Some of the patterns in serum concentration that may be expected from different regimens are shown in Figure 5.

The half-life of a drug is an important consideration in relation to the dosage interval. Generally speaking, if a drug is given at intervals that are substantially less than its half-life, it will accumulate. However, if the interval corresponds to the half-life, it will attain an equilibrium concentration after about four such doses. The steady-state concentration of a drug on different regimens can be calculated as shown in Figure 5.

It should be emphasized that although most drugs behave in a manner that allows such calculations and predictions to be made, there are

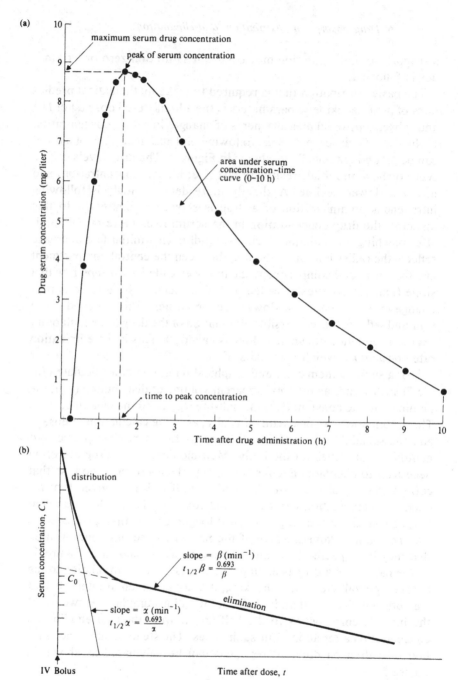

(a)

maximum serum drug concentration

peak of serum concentration

Drug serum concentration (mg/liter)

area under serum
concentration–time
curve (0–10 h)

time to peak concentration

Time after drug administration (h)

(b)

distribution

Serum concentration, C_1

slope $= \beta \, (\text{min}^{-1})$
$t_{1/2}\,\beta = \dfrac{0.693}{\beta}$

C_0

elimination

slope $= \alpha \, (\text{min}^{-1})$
$t_{1/2}\,\alpha = \dfrac{0.693}{\alpha}$

IV Bolus

Time after dose, t

Figure 4. (a) Serum concentration–time curve following oral administration of
hypothetical drugs. (From Koch-Weser, 1974a. Reprinted by permission from

36

Figure 5. Effects of varying doses and intervals between doses on drug accumulation during repeated administration. (a) The dose is varied, but the drug is administered at the same interval. (b) The interval between the dosages is varied, but the dose is kept constant. (c) When the dose is halved but is given twice as often, the steady-state concentration is maintained, but the fluctuation of the serum levels is reduced. (d) By administering an appropriate loading dose (1.5 to 2 times the maintenance dose), the steady-state serum concentration is achieved more rapidly. $t_{1/2}$, the half-life of the drug in the body; D, dose. (From Greenblatt and Koch-Weser, 1975b. Reprinted by permission from *The New England Journal of Medicine 293:967*)

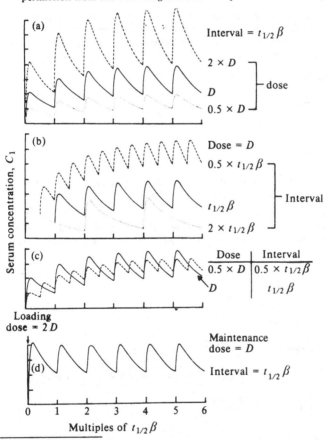

Caption to Fig. 4 (*cont.*)
The New England Journal of Medicine 291:234) (b) Graphic representation of the pharmacokinetic behavior of the serum concentration (C_1) of a drug following the injection of a single intravenous bolus. The predicted behavior follows that of the two-compartment open-model system (Figure 3b). The initial rapid decline (slope α) reflects the redistribution of the drug into its compartments. The subsequent slower elimination phase (slope β, or k_e) reflects its metabolism and excretion. The $t_{1/2}$ is the half-life of the drug with respect to its elimination (β). (From Greenblatt and Koch-Weser, 1975a. Reprinted by permission from *The New England Journal of Medicine 293:703*)

Table 5. *Some commonly used pharmacokinetic parameters of drugs*

Total absorbed dose or fractional absorption, f

$$f = \frac{\text{absorbed dose}}{\text{total administered dose } D}$$

$$f = \frac{\text{area under the curve (AUC) for time } (t) = \text{zero to } t = \infty \text{ after an oral or i.m. dose } (D)}{\text{AUC for } t = 0 \text{ to } t = \infty \text{ for i.v. dose } D}$$

The AUC is the area under the curve of serum drug concentration versus time. Its values provide relative information regarding the absorption of a drug following either different doses or administration via various routes (e.g., oral, intramuscular, subcutaneous, intravenous). The last is taken as the reference point, as in this case absorption is total.

Mathematically,

$$\text{AUC} = \frac{Df}{V_d k_e}$$

Total apparent volume of distribution, V_d

$$V_d = \frac{Df}{C_0} \text{ (liters)}$$

where C_0 is the serum concentration of the drug calculated from the intercept, at zero time, of the elimination curve (see Figure 3b)

Elimination rate constant, k_e
This value can be calculated from observed changes in the serum concentration of the drug during the elimination phase (Figure 3b). Its units are usually expressed as minutes.

Half-life for elimination, $t_{1/2}$ or $t_{1/2\beta}$

$$t_{1/2} = \frac{\ln 2}{k_e} = \frac{0.693}{k_e} \text{ (minutes)}$$

Clearance rate of a drug

$$\text{Clearance rate} = V_d \cdot k_e = \frac{V_d \cdot 0.693}{t_{1/2}} \text{ (liters/minute)}$$

Mean steady-state serum concentrations, C, with multiple doses of a drug

$$\bar{C} = \frac{1}{\text{clearance}} \cdot \frac{Df}{T} \text{ (mol/liter)}$$

or,

$$\frac{Df}{V_d k_e T} = \frac{1.44 \, Df t_{1/2}}{V_d T}$$

where T is the interval between doses, in minutes

These formulas can be transposed, as shown for $\bar{C}$, in various ways in accordance with the different methods for calculating the parameters or their individual terms. Other types of units can, of course, also be used. For more detailed information, see Greenblatt and Koch-Weser (1975a,b).

38

a number of notable exceptions. This problem may occur when the processes for elimination of a drug are saturable (they follow nonlinear or zero-order kinetics). The binding of drugs to plasma proteins, the formation of active metabolites, or persistent sequestration in other compartments, such as fat, can also complicate the use and interpretation of such pharmacokinetic methods.

7
The nature of responses to drugs

A drug ultimately acts to increase or decrease the activities of organs and cells. Such effects may be manifested in various ways, such as:

1. The contraction or relaxation of a muscle
2. An increase or decrease in the synthesis or release of a secretion (either exocrine or endocrine)
3. The uptake or loss of an ion (e.g., Na^+, K^+, Ca^{2+}) or metabolic substrate (e.g., a sugar, amino acid, or fatty acid)
4. The formation, activation, or degradation of an intracellular metabolite (e.g., cyclic AMP or GMP) or enzyme (e.g., RNA polymerase, adenyl cyclase, Na-K ATPase)
5. A change in the rate of growth, maturation, and division of cells

Such physiological processes are complex and invariably involve a number of sequential, but distinct, steps, each of which may provide a possible locus for interference by a drug. The responses are also usually dependent on the general integrity of the cell, so that an action of drugs on one type of process may indirectly influence another.

General requirements of a drug

A drug has several required general properties, which are dictated by its physicochemistry and the properties of its target tissues.

1. It should exhibit a propensity to react preferentially at certain tissue sites. This characteristic gives it a *selectivity* so that it can exert effects that are sufficiently specific to make it useful. Its side effects and toxicity are thus limited.
2. An ability to act at relatively low concentrations is usually desirable.
3. Its effects on the cell should generally be reversible so that permanent damage, which is difficult to repair, does not occur. However, covalent chemical interactions between certain drugs and tissues can be useful, such as in those compounds with chemotherapeutic cytotoxic actions.
4. Elimination from the body, as a result of its metabolism and/or excretion, must be possible.

How drugs act

Drugs act to alter the excitability and metabolic activities of tissues. They may elicit their effects on cells in several general ways, which can be placed in two main groups:

1. By reproducing, mimicking, or blocking the effects of natural excitants such as neurotransmitters and hormones. These effects may occur at any of a number of reaction sites that are involved in a response, such as an initial, terminal, or intermediate metabolic event.
2. By interfering with the normal formation, activation, degradation, or accumulation of natural metabolic substrates, enzymes, and ions.

Where drugs act in cells

Drugs usually act directly on their effector cells, but in some instances the initial site of their action may be elsewhere in the body. Thus, the activity of a tissue can be influenced by changes in its blood supply, the availability of external metabolites and ions such as glucose and Ca^{2+}, and stimulation by tropic hormones that are released into the circulation at some distal site.

Drugs may act at several different types of sites in cells:

1. They may act at the specific sites that normally mediate responses to natural excitants. Such natural receptors (see next section and Chapter 8) have been identified in the plasma membrane, the cytoplasm, and the nucleus, and may lie in close proximity or even be a component of enzymes. It seems likely that such receptors may also be associated with other parts of cells, such as storage granules, mitochondria, and the Golgi apparatus.
2. Changes may occur as a result of a generalized physicochemical interaction with structural components of the cell, especially the various membranes that sequester its contents. Such changes may alter the intracellular distribution of ions and metabolites and so evoke responses, including changes in muscular contractility and secretion. These interactions may occur at localized specific sites, such as the action of tetrodotoxin, which blocks sodium channels in nerve and muscle membranes. The effect may, however, be a very general one that need not have precise structural requirements but simply involves the saturation of a biophase of the cell such as the membrane lipids (a phenomenon called the Ferguson principle). Many anesthetics appear to act in this manner.
3. A physical or chemical interaction with tissue enzymes and metabolic substrates may occur that alters their structural conformation and ability to take part in the normal processes in the cell. This may involve the substitution of a "fake" metabolite that can enter the system but will not undergo normal transformation. An interaction

with an allosteric enzyme may change its conformation and initiate a response.

   Receptors were originally hypothetical components of cells, the existence of which was proposed to account for the actions of drugs and natural physiological excitants present in the body. Over the last few years their presence has received dramatic confirmation (see Ariëns, 1979) as a result of the precise physicochemical identification of a number of such receptors, especially those for hormones and neurotransmitters, in tissues and extracts of cells. The term receptors has on occasion been used to describe any physical or chemical site with which a drug, neurotransmitter, or hormone can react in the cell. Such a definition is, however, now too broad to be useful and does not fulfill the requirements of the original receptor hypothesis. The term receptor is at present generally reserved for specific natural sites that are present at low concentrations in cells. Such distinct components can be viewed as having been formed as a result of the normal processes of evolution and may even be considered as another type of cellular organelle, but they are only of molecular (or macromolecular) dimensions and usually exist as a part of, or in close association with, larger structures. Some receptors, however, have been "solubilized" and separated from other parts of the cell.

   The existence of such a receptor for a drug suggests the presence of natural homologues to the drug with which it combines, although these have not always been identified. A dramatic example of such a relationship has, however, been provided by the identification of natural substances that can combine with "opiate receptors." The actions of the opiate drugs morphine and heroin have been known for hundreds of years, and recently specific receptors for them were isolated from brain and intestine. Subsequently, starting in 1975, a group of naturally occurring peptides, the enkephalins and endorphins, that react with these opiate receptors, were isolated from brain tissue. Up-to-date summaries of information about peptide and steroid hormone receptors have been provided by O'Malley and Schrader (1976), Catt and Dufau (1977), and Hollenberg and Cuatrecasas (1978).

The role of receptors

The function of receptors in the body is to sort out information that may be provided to the cells by the blood and nerves that supply them, and, when appropriate, to transmit a signal to the machinery of the cells. A receptor thus acts as a transducer. The energy provided by such an initial signal is usually very small compared to that involved in the final response; so the receptor also plays a role in the process of amplification that is necessary for a full response to occur. It should be emphasized that responses to drugs are usually quite complex and may involve a whole series of reactions in which the interaction with the receptor is quite distal to the ultimate response. That interaction is still an essential, primary event, however.

8
Receptor theory

Drugs and hormones usually act at relatively low concentrations, frequently at about 10^{-9} M, although concentrations as low as 10^{-12} M are not uncommon. Their effects are also usually remarkably specific in relation to their chemical structure. Specific properties of drugs have been recognized for about 100 years, and led J. N. Langley in 1905 to suggest the presence of a specific "receptive substance" to account for the actions of curare and nicotine at the neuromuscular junction. P. Ehrlich made a similar suggestion in 1913 to explain the specific actions of certain dyes on bacteria. Although receptors remained somewhat enigmatic hypothetical entities until quite recently, they provided a basis for the theoretical analysis of the quantitative actions of drugs, both in eliciting a response (agonists) and in antagonizing it (antagonists). Several such theories to account for the actions of drugs have been proposed. The two major current ones are the *occupation theory*, originally developed about 50 years ago by A. J. Clark at University College London, and the *rate theory*, proposed by W. D. M. Paton at Oxford in 1961 (Paton, 1961). Occupation theory has been somewhat modified, especially by E. J. Ariëns (see Ariëns and Simonis, 1964a,b), and is currently the more favored one. It should, however, be emphasized that no single theory can completely account for all the various phenomena associated with drug action, and it is possible that some groups of drugs act differently, so that a unitary theory may not be appropriate. In addition, conclusive experimental proof of such theories is probably not feasible, although they can provide a useful and productive framework for understanding the mechanisms by which drugs work.

Occupation theory

When the concentration of a drug is plotted in relation to its response, such as the contraction of a piece of smooth muscle in an organ bath,

44

there is a rapid rise in the effects, once the threshold level has been achieved, in relation to the increasing level of the drug. Eventually, saturation occurs, and a hyperbolic curve is seen (Figure 6a). Such a dose–response relationship is also frequently plotted using a logarithmic scale for the dose or concentration, and this gives a sigmoidal-shaped curve (Figure 6b). (The latter has certain practical advantages, as the central part of the curve is linear, which facilitates comparisons of the potency of drugs.) Clark proposed that the effects of a drug were proportional to the quantity of the receptor–drug complex, so that when the response is 50 percent of maximal, half of the receptors are bound to the drug. (As we shall see, this half-saturation is an oversimplification, as maximal responses can often be obtained when only a small proportion of the total receptors present are occupied.) Such a relationship can be described in terms of the law of mass action. Thus, according to the mass action law:

$$[\text{drug}] + [\text{receptor}] \underset{k_2}{\overset{k_1}{\rightleftharpoons}} [\text{drug–receptor complex}]$$

where k_1 and k_2 are the rate constants for the forward and backward reactions, respectively. The ratio k_2/k_1, or

$$\frac{[\text{drug}] \times [\text{receptor}]}{[\text{drug–receptor complex}]}$$

is called the equilibrium dissociation constant K_d, K_{diss}, or most often K_D, although the term K_A is also used for an agonist drug. K_D is expressed in moles per liter and is expected to be equivalent to the concentration of the drug that is present when the response is 50 percent of the maximum (ED50) attainable by that drug. Such an analysis of hormone–receptor interactions is analogous to that used to describe the combination of enzymes with their substrates, in which case the equilibrium constant k_2/k_1 is K_m (the Michaelis-Menton constant). The equilibrium association constant k_1/k_2 can also be used to describe this reaction. It is expressed as K_a or K_s and has units of liters per mole.

Affinity and intrinsic activity

Drugs interact with their receptors with differing degrees of readiness or strength, and the attractive property of a drug is called its *affinity* for its receptor. Affinity is inversely proportional to the dissociation constant ($1/K_D$ or K_a), so that affinity is said to be high if the concentration of a drug that results in 50 percent saturation of the receptors is low. The affinity is also expressed as PD_2, which is the negative logarithm of the molar concentration producing a half-maximal response. Thus, if this concentration is 10^{-9} M, the PD_2 is 9. The higher the value, the greater the affinity the drug has for its receptor.

Different drugs, even when they are closely related chemically, can exhibit quite different abilities to elicit a response, and some may even act as antagonists. Such properties cannot be readily accounted for simply in terms of the law of mass action, and it was proposed that drugs have other properties related to the strength of the effect they can elicit. Stephenson referred to the *efficacy* of a drug, and Ariëns termed this property *intrinsic activity* (α):

$$\text{response} = \alpha \ (\text{drug–receptor complex})$$

Alpha is a proportionality constant related to the drug's intrinsic ability to elicit a response once it has combined with the receptor. In terms of the law of mass action, it can be described as

$$\text{drug} + \text{receptor} \underset{k_2}{\overset{k_1}{\rightleftharpoons}} \text{drug–receptor complex}$$

$$\xrightarrow{k_3} \text{receptor} + \text{response}$$

In enzyme kinetics, k_3 is the rate constant of the final step of the reaction; in the present analogy it is equivalent to the intrinsic activity.

Figure 6. Drug concentration or dose–response curves. (a) The response, plotted as a percent of the maximal one (= 100 percent) versus the drug concentration. The curve has a hyperbolic shape. At a response equivalent to 50 percent of the maximal one (ED50), receptor "occupation theory" predicts that 50 percent of the receptors will be occupied. The concentration of the drug at which this occurs will then be expected to be equivalent to K_D or, by analogy with enzyme (for the drug–receptor interaction) kinetics, K_m. (b) The dose of the drug is more often plotted in relation to the logarithm of its concentration, so that a sigmoidal-shaped curve is seen. For further details see text.

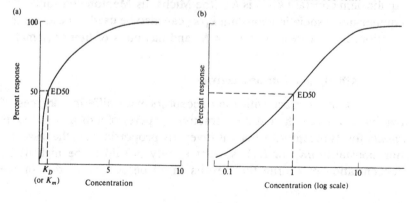

The efficacy or intrinsic activity of a drug is the maximal or ceiling effect that it can elicit. Different members of a group of drugs may differ in their ability to bring about such a response, but the one that exerts the highest effect ever observed is said to have an intrinsic activity of 1. Plotted graphically, this can be seen to correspond to the 100 percent response. A drug that can elicit only 50 percent of this maximal response has an α of 0.5. The affinity ($1/K_D$) may or may not be the same for drugs with differing intrinsic activities.

Intrinsic activity should not be equated with *potency*, which is a comparison of the abilities of drugs to elicit the same quantitative response. It can be seen in Figure 7 that when we compare the abilities of the three drugs to elicit the same response, for instance, equivalent to 50 percent of the maximum response, A and B have similar potencies (despite their quite different intrinsic activities), whereas C is about four times less potent. It can be seen that the ED50 (the dose or concentration giving a half-maximal response, also described as the A_{50}) and

Figure 7. Intrinsic activities (α) and affinities ($1/K_D$) of three drugs as illustrated from their concentration–percent response curves. The maximal responses differ in all three drugs, so that they have intrinsic activities of 1, 0.75, and 0.5. The affinities ($1/K_D$) for each drug do not, however, necessarily have the same relative relationship. In this instance drug B displays the greatest affinity for its receptor. This figure also illustrates the difficulties of predicting the potency of a drug from either its intrinsic activity or its affinity. Thus, if a response corresponding to 25 percent of the maximal one were chosen for comparison, drugs A and B would have the same potency, and they would be about four times as potent as drug C. However, at 75 percent maximal response, drug A would clearly be the most potent.

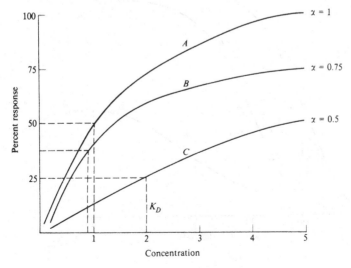

thus the affinities ($1/K_D$) of each drug for its receptor, are in this instance different. (ED50 is also not necessarily related to potency.)

Some of these relationships, especially those of affinity, are seen more clearly when such results are plotted as the logarithm of the dose (Figure 8). In this instance, drugs A and B have the same intrinsic activity (α), but 10 times more B is needed to elicit the same response (it is 10 times less potent). C requires 10 to 1000 times the dose of A, depending on which point in the two nonparallel curves one chooses to make the comparison. It can be seen that although drugs A and B can elicit the same maximal response, the plot for B is displaced in parallel to the right. The ED50 is 10 times greater, so that its affinity ($1/K_D$) for its receptor is much less than that of A. This type of difference, where two drugs have the same intrinsic activity but differing affinities, is usually seen in drugs that are structurally related and suggests that they are probably interacting with the same receptor. (There are, how-

Figure 8. Relationships of affinity, intrinsic activity, and potency of three drugs A, B, and C. The concentration is plotted on a log scale. Drugs A and B have the same intrinsic activity ($\alpha = 1$), but the dose–response curve for B is displaced in parallel to the right, so that the K_D for its drug–receptor complex appears to be 10 times greater. (It has a lower affinity for the receptor.) In this instance, drug B is also 10 times less potent than drug A. Drug C has a lower intrinsic activity (= 0.5) than drugs A and B, and the dose–response curve is displaced far to the right and is not parallel to the other curves. Although it would appear that drugs A and B are chemically related to each other, drug C is probably quite different from drugs A and B.

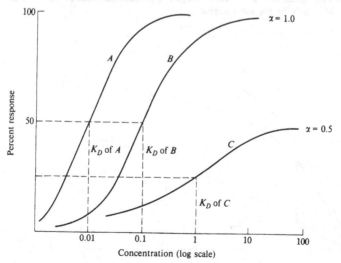

ever, exceptions, and this likelihood is not a rule.) Drug C is quite different from A and B, as it not only has a lower intrinsic activity, but its ED50, and hence K_D, corresponds to the log dose of 1. Its dose–response plot is not only displaced far to the right, but in contrast to drugs A and B it is not parallel to the other curves. These observations indicate that C is not acting in the same way as are A and B, and its structure will almost certainly be quite different from those of A and B.

Antagonism

Drugs are widely used to antagonize the effects of other drugs and endogenous physiological responses such as those to neurotransmitters and hormones. They may exert such effects in various ways, including an opposing physiological response, such as activating the relaxation as opposed to the contraction of a muscle (physiological antagonism). Antagonists may also work more specifically by exerting an effect on the same response mechanism (pharmacological antagonism). As already described, the response to an excitant may be quite a complex process and involve numerous individual but related sequential effects. Thus, it is feasible to block such an effect of a drug at various points. In the instance of smooth muscle contraction, this effect could involve the release of a neurotransmitter, a drug's access to or interaction with its receptor, the membrane depolarization process, coupling events that involve an increase in cytoplasmic Ca^{2+}, or the activity of the contractile proteins themselves. An endocrine example would be the events that result in the antidiuretic effect of vasopressin (antidiuretic hormone, ADH), which includes an interaction with its receptor, activation of adenyl cyclase, synthesis and destruction of cyclic AMP, activation of a protein kinase, and the integrity of the actual mechanism that increases the permeability of the renal tubular cells to water.

Dose–response curves to a drug are plotted in Figure 9 in relation to the presence of different concentrations of two types of antagonists. It can be seen that when the excitant drug E, an agonist, is present with drug A (an antagonist), the response is depressed, but, provided that the concentration of E is raised enough, the same effect can be elicited. In the log dose–response plot, the curve for E + drug A is displaced in parallel to the right. This form of antagonism is the *competitive* type. In its simplest interpretation, in terms of receptor theory, drugs E and A may be considered as competing for the same receptor, a situation that

Figure 9. Drug dose–response curves, illustrating competitive and noncompetitive antagonism. Two types of plots are made using an arithmetic (a) and a log concentration (b) scale. It can be seen in both (a) and (b) that when a fixed concentration of drug A (an antagonist) is administered at the same time as drug E (the excitant or agonist), a higher concentration of E must be used to elicit the same effect as A. Provided that enough of E is administered, however, the same maximal response can be achieved. The antagonism can be overcome and is said to be competitive. In the instance of the second antagonist, drug B, however, the decrease in the effect cannot be overcome; its effect is insurmountable or noncompetitive.

(a)

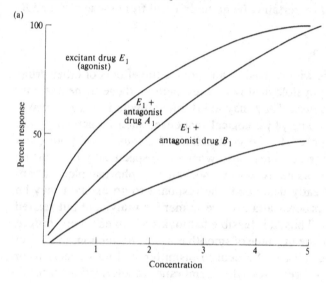

(b)

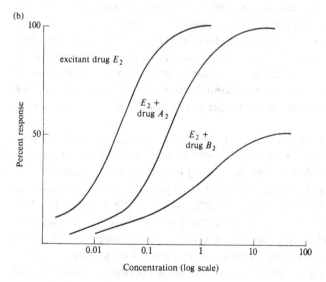

most likely reflects similarities in their structures. A change in the conformation of the receptor that reduces its affinity for the drug may also be occurring in the presence of the antagonist. It is difficult to exclude the possibility that the antagonist may be influencing a more distal process in the chain of the effector response, the rate of which is closely related to the primary drug–receptor interaction. In this instance, however, the two drugs would probably be structurally dissimilar (remarkable coincidences excepted). Competitive antagonists are considered to have an affinity for the receptor but a low, or zero, intrinsic activity. They may still (although usually at relatively high concentrations) elicit responses themselves, and are then called *partial agonists*, but they can usually produce only submaximal responses.

The antagonism of drug B for drug E (Figure 9) is quite different from that of A for E. In this instance, no matter how much the concentration of E is increased, its original response cannot be restored; the antagonism is insurmountable. This is called *noncompetitive antagonism*. A displacement of the response to the right can be seen in the log dose–response plot, but it is not parallel to the original effect of E. The effects of such an antagonist may occur at some rate-limiting step of the response, distal to the drug–receptor complex. It remains possible, however, that the latter is affected in some way, as would happen, for example, if the antagonist combined with some adjacent moiety, and so excluded the drug from its receptor. The formation of an irreversible covalent linkage to the receptor or some other form of receptor inactivation is also expected to result in this type of effect (but not if there are "spare" receptors; see next paragraph).

As emphasized at the beginning of this section, the occupation theory cannot account for all observations on the responses of tissues to drugs. Various modifications have therefore been proposed, one of the most important of them being the concept of *receptor reserve* or *spare receptors,* which was made necessary by several types of observations. On the basis of occupation theory, as originally proposed, the log dose-response curves should have a slope of unity, but in many instances this is not observed. The slope is often much steeper than this (see Rang, 1971). It has also been observed that whereas certain drugs (notable the β-haloalkylamines, which are α-adrenergic inhibitors) that covalently bind to receptors, and so irreversibly inactivate them, result in a decline in the maximal response at high concentrations, at lower levels they simply produce a parallel displacement of the curve to the right. Thus under the latter condition, a maximal response can still be attained, although with higher levels of the agonist. This effect would not be possible if 100 percent of the receptors were required to elicit the full effect. These observations led to the suggestion that, in fact, not all the receptors need to be occupied, and that in some instances only a small percentage need to combine with the drug in order to elicit the normal maximal response. Thus, there may be an excess or reserve in the numbers of receptors. More direct counts of receptors have recently been obtained for several hormone-responsive tissues, and the relationship of their occupancy to the response has confirmed this theory of spare receptors.

The potency of an antagonist can be expressed as the pA_2, as described by Schild (1957). This value is the negative logarithm of the concentration of the antagonist, which requires a doubling of the concentration of the agonist to overcome its inhibitory effects. The higher the value, the more effective the antagonist (pA_{10} values are also sometimes used).

Rate theory

Although most observations on drug–receptor interactions are consistent with the action of a drug being elicited while it actually occupies a site on the receptor, this cannot account for all such phenomena. In addition, as we have seen, the occupation theory has been modified in several ways, especially with the introduction of the concept of intrinsic activity to account for the fact that occupancy of a receptor can have either an agonistic or an antagonistic effect. Other basic problems arise when one tries to explain how some drugs (e.g., nicotine) first stimulate and then block a response. Many drugs also initially exert an effect that subsequently declines, or "fades," even though the drug remains in contact with the tissue.

In 1961, Paton presented a theory to account for such anachronisms, which he called *rate theory*. It was proposed that excitation of the receptor only occurs in a quantal manner as a result of its initial combination, or collision, with the drug. Further effects are dependent on its ability to dissociate from the receptor so that it is free to be stimulated once again. It is therefore the rate of stimulation or number of successful collisions of the drug with its receptor that is important in eliciting a response. In terms of association (k_1) and dissociation (k_2) rate constants of the reaction

$$[\text{drug}] + [\text{receptor}] \underset{k_2}{\overset{k_1}{\rightleftharpoons}} [\text{drug–receptor complex}]$$

an effective agonist must also have a high k_2, whereas an antagonist will have a low k_2 and will so limit the rate of new collisions. The k_2 or rate of dissociation of the drug–receptor complex thus determines what in occupation theory is called the intrinsic activity, whereas the affinity remains equivalent to the reciprocal of the dissociation constant k_2/k_1 ($1/K_D$). Stimulation followed by blockade or fading of a response can be accounted for by the difficulty that a drug may have in dissociating from its drug–receptor complex following the initial successful collision that produces an effect. Clearly, rate theory has its attractions despite the current popularity of occupation theory.

Physicochemical nature of the interaction of a drug and its receptor

To trigger a biological response a drug must not only interact with a receptor, but must do so in a manner that is sufficiently favorable to elicit or fulfill any change that may be required by the receptor. It is clear that most receptors have very specific requirements, as what appear to be quite small changes in the structure of a drug can result in dramatic changes in its activity. Thus, one form of a drug may be highly effective, whereas a stereoisomer of it may completely lack the ability to interact with a receptor. In other instances, some form of interaction between a drug and receptor may occur, but it may only elicit a partial response or even none at all. The precise reasons for such differences are not completely understood, but it is suspected that they ultimately could reflect the nature of the alignment, or stereochemical fit, and chemical interactions between the drug and its receptor. A favorable collision and combination most often appear to depend on a physicochemical interaction involving several sites on the molecules, those on the drug being complementary to those on the receptor. In some instances, such as those involving complex polypeptides, such interacting sites may be quite numerous.

Probably the primary requirement for a drug's success in combining with a receptor is its three-dimensional shape or conformation (tertiary structure). This may be important for several reasons.

1. The drug's route to its receptor site is sometimes conceived of as occurring through a specifically shaped cavity, such as a cleft or pore.
2. The receptor itself is also thought to have an intricate three-dimensional shape which may be complementary to the drug, so that the two fit into each other like a pair of oddly shaped wooden blocks.
3. Probably of more basic importance, however, is the fact that the shape of the drug molecule will determine the respective positions and

alignments, and even the existence, of the various forces that are necessary for its successful interaction with its receptor. These areas of force may not only be present individually on the receptor and drug, but may also be induced following their alignment as a result, for example, of dipole–dipole interactions between them. The approach and proximity of two such molecules can result in changes in both of them, including alterations in their conformation.

The lipid and water solubility of a drug may also be important, and may determine its ability to gain access to the region of its receptor. This will be influenced by such factors as the presence and distribution of polar and nonpolar chemical groups and the degree of ionization of the molecule at the ambient pH (its pK_a). (Ionized drugs are much less lipid-soluble; see Chapter 10).

Several types of forces may be involved in the interactions of drugs and receptors, and several of them may take part in the formation of a single drug–receptor complex. The irreversible *covalent-type bond* is not typically involved, although it does occur and, as with the α-adrenergic blocker phenoxybenzamine or the cholinesterase inhibitor DFP, usually results in an inhibitory-type response. Certain cytotoxic antineoplastic drugs, which, for instance, bind to components in the nucleus, also interact with tissues irreversibly. Toxic drugs and metabolites often bind covalently to tissues. Such responses and interactions are difficult to reverse and may depend on the normal processes of tissue replacement and growth. Weaker electrostatic forces are more usual and result in the reversible type of interactions that are essential for a receptor's normal activity. These forces may be simple *ionic bonds* which are provided by carboxyl (—COOH) or phosphoryl (—OPO$_3$H$_2$) moieties and by partially ionized sulfhydryl (—SH) groups. Cationic sites include the guanidinium moiety such as is present on arginine, the ϵ-ammonium on lysine, and partially ionized terminal α-ammonium (—NH$_2^+$) and amide (—CONH$_2$) groups on glutamine. Hydroxyl groups on a phenolic or aromatic structure are not ionized at a physiological pH.

When the drug and receptor are in close proximity to each other, short-range, relatively weak electrical forces can operate, as a result of *attraction between dipoles*. Dipoles arise because of disparities in the distribution of electrons between two adjacent sites, such as the carbon and the oxygen in the carbonyl (C=O) group (the oxygen is more electronegative). The close proximity of two electron-dense regions in separate molecules may also be sufficient to produce a redistribution of electrons so that an induced dipole (*van der Waals forces*) is formed. Such dipoles, utilizing either their cationic or anionic sites, can interact (dipole–dipole interactions) with a complementary adjacent charge and so contribute to a link between two molecules.

Hydrogen bonds are commonly utilized in drug–receptor inter-actions. Hydrogen can form cross-linkages between two partially negative electron-rich sites, both within molecules and between molecules. They can thus link peptide groups ($\diagdown$C=O $\cdots$ H—N$\diagup$),

hydroxyls (C$\diagup$ OH $\cdots$ O$\diagdown$$\overset{\text{H}}{\diagup}$ C$\diagdown$), or carboxy and hydroxy moieties.

Hydrophobic forces appear to be frequently involved in the interac-tion of drugs and receptors. In aqueous solutions, both drug and recep-tor are usually surrounded by a halo of ordered water molecules. In-teractions between hydrophobic groups in the drug and receptor result in the release of water molecules as the two molecules approach each other, and the release of water molecules results in an increase in the entropy (disorderliness) of the system that drives the reaction forward. The free energy of the receptor–drug system will thus be lowered as compared to that of its separated components in solution. Their aggre-gation will thus be favored, and this, predominantly entropic, effect is referred to as a hydrophobic interaction.

Identification of receptors

The direct identification of specific receptors for drugs, and hormones, depends on the use of radioactively labelled compounds that have a high specific activity (i.e., radioactivity per mole of drug or hormone). Such substances, when labelled in the more usual way with ^{125}I or ^{3}H, should retain their biological activity. Tissues, usually studied in vitro, but also in vivo, can be shown to accumulate such compounds, but as this process may involve several types of sites, it is necessary to distin-guish specific binding such as would be expected to occur to receptors, from nonspecific binding that occurs elsewhere in the tissue. To make this distinction, the tissue is exposed to a relatively low concentration of the labelled drug or hormone, and, after a period of time is allowed for equilibration, an excess (usually about 1000 times greater concentration) of the unlabelled "cold" material is added. This procedure is expected to displace the labelled drug from its specific binding sites and to give a measure of the receptors. This effect is shown in Figure 10, in which ^{125}I-insulin is displaced from binding to rat liver cell membranes. In this instance, only about 10 percent of the bound insulin was present at nonspecific sites. In many instances, however, this nonspecific fraction may be much greater and even the predominant one. It can be seen (in Figure 10) that other polypeptide hormones, such as corticotropin (ACTH), glucagon, and growth hormone, did not displace the ^{125}I-insulin from binding. Bovine and human insulin were as effective as

Figure 10. Identification of "specific" receptor sites for insulin on rat liver membranes. These preparations were exposed to labelled porcine ^{125}I-insulin at a concentration of 0.7 nM (4 ng/ml). The radioactivity in the pellet of the membrane preparation is then plotted as a function of "cold" unlabelled hormone preparations. It can be seen that ACTH, glucagon, and human growth hormone (hGH) failed to alter the amount of radioactivity in the pellet, but three different preparations of insulin (human, bovine, and porcine) all displaced radioactivity from binding to the membrane preparations. This displaced radioactivity is considered to correspond to that which is specifically bound, most probably to the insulin receptors. With a 1000-fold excess of "cold" insulin, it can be seen that only about 10 percent of the originally bound material is still present, which corresponds to "nonspecific" binding. (From Freychet et al., 1971)

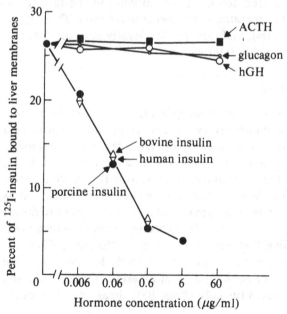

"cold" porcine insulin in displacing the bound (labelled) porcine insulin. However, insulins from other species or modified preparations (analogues) or the separated A- or B-chains of the hormone were less effective, reflecting their relative abilities to combine with the receptors in the rat liver membranes (Figure 11, top graph). These differences in affinity for the receptors can also be seen to be reflected in their biological responses (stimulation of glucose oxidation in fat cells; Figure 11, bottom graph). Such structural specificity for the binding sites and the quantitative relationship of this association to the biological response are important criteria in confirming that such sites are really the receptors.

As receptor sites are expected to be finite in number, they should be saturable with the drug or hormone. An example of this property, using ^{125}I-human growth hormone, is shown in Figure 12. It can be seen that specific binding of this hormone to rat liver membranes can be detected at about 10 pmol/liter and reaches saturation at 360 pmol/liter. Nonspecific binding of the hormones, however, did not display saturation at these concentrations.

A receptor is expected to have a high affinity constant ($1/K_D$) for a drug or hormone. This value can be estimated in several ways, including calculation from dose–response curves of the concentration at which 50 percent saturation of the receptors occurs. In 1949, G. Scatchard described a theoretical way of estimating the affinity of proteins for small molecules, as well as the number of sites on the protein that are occupied. This involves plotting the ratio bound/free molecules (e.g., a drug or hormone) on the ordinate, and plotting on the abscissa the amount that is bound. The intercept with the abscissa gives an estimate of the number of binding sites, and the slope indicates the affinity. An example that involves the binding of [^{3}H]aldosterone to toad bladder tissue (a model for the kidney) is shown in Figure 13. It can be seen that two groups of binding sites can be distinguished, one with a high affinity but with a relatively small number of sites and the other with a lower affinity but more numerous binding sites. Estimates of numbers of receptors per cell depend on the particular system being studied, but vary from about 1000 to more than 100,000.

Using such modern techniques for studying and isolating receptors, it is now possible to define such values as the equilibrium dissociation constant, K_D, of the drug–receptor complex by direct measurements. Thus, the concentration that corresponds to 50 percent saturation of the binding of a drug, or hormone, to its specific receptors is the K_D (some-

58

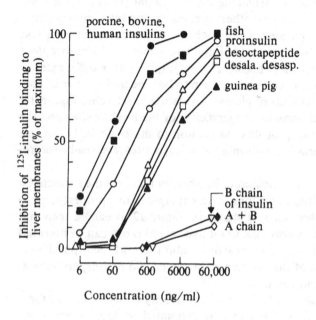

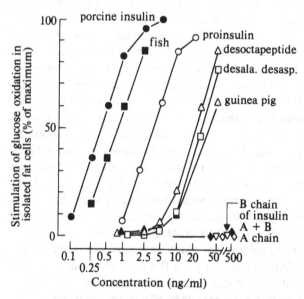

Figure 11. Parallel abilities of different insulin preparations to bind to receptors and to elicit a biological response. As shown in Figure 10, specific binding of insulin to rat liver membrane preparations can be measured by recording their abilities to displace porcine ^{125}I-insulin from specific binding receptor sites. Whereas the receptors in the rat liver membrane preparations (top graph) apparently cannot distinguish between human, porcine, and bovine insulin, it

Figure 12. Saturation of the specific binding sites for ^{125}I-human growth hormone to rat liver membranes (●). In contrast, it can be seen that at the concentration used, nonspecific binding (o) did not display such saturation. (From Herington et al., 1976)

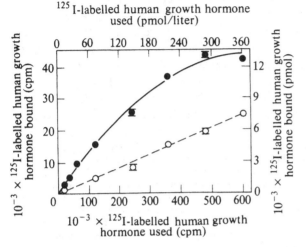

^{125}I-labelled human growth hormone used (pmol/liter)

$10^{-3} \times$ ^{125}I-labelled human growth hormone used (cpm)

times called K_D binding). This determination involves measurements of the ability of unlabelled drug to displace labelled drug from its receptor sites. If, however, a suitable labelled form of the drug is not available, then this parameter can be obtained by measuring its ability to displace a labelled analogue from binding. This value is the same as the K_i, the inhibition equilibrium constant for an antagonist. It is the concentration necessary to displace 50 percent of the bound (labelled) drug. As described earlier, such values as the K_D, as well as the K_i, can be estimated less directly by recording, respectively, the concentrations necessary to elicit a half-maximal response or to inhibit a maximal response by 50 percent. Such values are sometimes called the $K_{D\text{ apparent}}$ ($K_{D\text{ app}}$) or the $K_{D\text{ activation}}$ ($K_{D\text{ act}}$). The measured biological response may be that of a final effector, such as the contraction of a piece of smooth muscle, or it can involve an intermediate type of response,

Caption to Fig. 11 (cont.)
may be seen that fish and guinea pig insulin, proinsulin, and chemically modified fragments (desoctapeptide and desalanine, desaspartic acid–insulin, as well as the separated A- and B-insulin chains) are much less effective in displacing the porcine insulin. In the bottom graph it can be seen that the biological response (stimulation of glucose oxidation) by fat cells displayed a parallel responsiveness to the receptor binding of the different preparations of insulin. (From Freychet et al., 1971)

such as the activation of an enzyme that is involved, such as adenyl cyclase. The two values of the K_D determined in these ways ($K_{D\,binding}$ and $K_{D\,activation}$) do not always correspond. The possible reasons for this behavior include the presence of spare receptors, in which case only a small proportion of the total may need to be activated to elicit a maximal response. It has also been viewed (Maguire et al., 1977) as reflecting differences in the coupling efficiency between the drug–receptor complex and the response – for instance, activation of adenylate cyclase. If the ratio $K_{D\,binding}/K_{D\,activation}$ is greater than 1, it suggests that relatively few receptors may need to be occupied to activate each unit of the effector substance (e.g., an enzyme). The converse could occur if

Figure 13. Scatchard plot of the binding of [³H]aldosterone to toad urinary bladder in vitro. This preparation is commonly used to study the actions of hormones and drugs on the kidney. When plotted in this way, the binding of the aldosterone indicates that there are two sets of binding sites. The intercepts with the abscissa indicate the maximal numbers of each of these, whereas the slopes of the lines reflect the affinity of the aldosterone for each set of the receptors. It can be seen that the receptors indicated by the first part of the line are less numerous but have a higher affinity for the hormone than the others. (From Sharp et al., 1966)

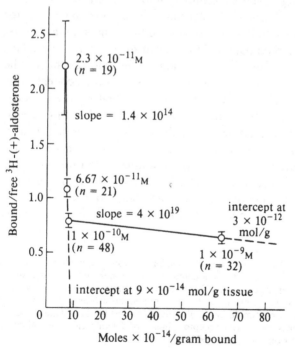

activation of multiple receptors were involved in triggering the activation of each such enzyme unit.

Such methods for identifying and counting receptors and the theoretical analysis of the results are not without criticisms and constraints. Some of these have been reviewed by Cuatrecasas et al. (1975). The original analysis of the molecular binding process which was performed by Scatchard involved soluble proteins and relatively small molecules that were bound with a low affinity. The process of drug and hormone receptor interactions usually differs somewhat from the process described by Scatchard. The distinction between specific and nonspecific binding can also sometimes be difficult and depends on the conditions, including the concentrations used and even the amount of shaking and the nature of the containers in which the reaction is studied. What appears to be specific binding can occur on the walls of cellulose acetate tubes and Millipore filters. Insulin can even be shown to bind to talc in a manner suggesting the presence of a specific receptor. Thus, the process of adsorption can imitate the binding of a drug or hormone to its receptor. Clearly, the identification and measurement of receptors requires, apart from theoretical knowledge, considerable experience, critical ability, and a sense of skepticism.

Nature of receptors

In 1960, Schueler described a receptor in physical terms as follows: "The drug–receptor is in general the pattern R of forces of diverse origin forming a part of some biological system and having roughly the same dimensions as a certain pattern M of forces presented by the drug molecule in such a way that between patterns M and R a relationship of complementarity for interaction exists" (p. 140). This concept is still valid, but today we have available more concrete information about the factors that determine these properties.

The availability of radioactively labelled drugs and hormones has facilitated the direct study of receptors (see preceding section). An important technical advance was the utilization of the principles of radioimmunoassays for competitive-binding studies. Receptors in various tissues and organs have been studied, using such methods, both in vitro and in vivo. Cell fractionation procedures have also been utilized to identify and study receptors in the microsomes, cytoplasm, and nuclei of cells. Soluble receptors that are normally present in the cytoplasm have been isolated, and in some instances those that are present in the plasma membrane have been solubilized with the aid of detergents such as Triton-X.

The receptors for hormones, which are also often occupied by drugs, have provided the most dramatic advances in our knowledge of these constituents of cells. They are proteinaceous and usually have a molecular weight of about 60,000 to 300,000 and a hydrodynamic radius of 60 to 70 Å. Some of these receptors have been shown to be oligomeric and contain subunits, each of which may or may not bind an excitant molecule. Their protein nature is reflected in their sensitivity to proteolytic enzymes such as trypsin and to SH-reactive chemicals. Some hormone receptors have been shown to contain carbohydrate moieties and are thus probably glycoproteins. The properties of some receptors that are attached to membranes are altered following incubation with phospholipase enzymes. This observation may reflect the nature of their association with the plasma membrane, or they may contain a lipid component that is essential for their activity.

Steroid hormones and their drug analogues have been shown to bind to receptors, or "acceptors," in the nucleus (see Figure 14). These nuclear receptors are present in the chromatin, where they are associated with acidic, nonhistone proteins. To interact with these nuclear receptors, the steroid must, it appears, first be bound to the cytoplasmic receptor, which helps to effect its transfer into the nucleus and the binding process. Steroids can bind to naked nuclear DNA, but this process is not specific.

Receptors have a high degree of specificity with respect to the structure of the molecule they can combine with; stereoisomers of a drug usually cannot bind to the receptor. Usually, a receptor only binds one molecule of an agonist or antagonist, but in some instances, such as certain cytoplasmic steroid hormone receptor subunits, more than one molecule may be bound.

Receptors have high affinity (a K_D of about 10^{-8} to 10^{-11}) for their ligands. The interactions may depend on various external factors, including the pH and the presence of divalent ions, especially Ca^{2+} and Mg^{2+}. Such ions may alter the affinity of the receptor for a drug, possibly by altering its conformation.

Membrane receptors are thought to consist of a hydrophobic base associated with the lipids in which it lies and a hydrophilic apex that projects into the external aqueous solution. Their position or function may be related to the cell microfilament system, as in some instances the cytochalasin drugs can block their functioning. It is considered that receptors either may have a relatively fixed position in the plasma membrane, or they may be able to move about laterally in it ("mobile receptor theory"). Either type of receptor is expected to have a spatial relationship, either fixed or flexible, to another membrane component that helps relay its signal. In the instance of many polypeptide hormones and catecholamines, this constituent is adenylate cyclase (see also Chapter 10). This enzyme system is thought to contain at least two other important components, apart from the receptor: a *catalytic site*, which is concerned with its interaction with ATP, and a *regulatory site*, which controls the conformation of the enzyme by its ability to combine with nucleotides, mainly GTP, and possibly also to alter the drug–receptor interaction.

By labelling hormones and their antibodies with radioactive atoms or fluorescent compounds, it has been possible to trace their distribution following their interaction with cells. It has recently become apparent the "membrane" receptors are not necessarily confined to the plasma membrane. Various large polypeptides, including insulin, growth hor-

Figure 14. General mechanism of the action of sex steroid hormones as constructed by Chan and O'Malley (1976). This scheme was composed principally on information gathered from studies on the progesterone receptor in the chick oviduct. S, steroid hormone; R_A and R_B, the subunits of the steroid hormone receptors. (From Chan and O'Malley, 1976. Reprinted by permission from *The New England Journal of Medicine 294:*1322)

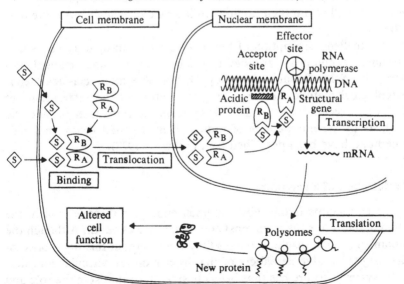

mone, and prolactin, have been identified, following a period of incubation, within cells (see Kolata, 1978). Specific receptor sites for such hormones have also been identified associated with the Golgi apparatus. The mechanism and function of this entry of the hormone into the cell are not clear. It seems likely that it brings its membrane receptor with it, and this could involve a process of endocytosis following aggregation in areas called "coated pits" (Goldstein et al., 1979). Functionally, this process could provide a method for inactivating a hormone or a drug regulating the number of membrane receptors. It is also feasible that such "internalized" hormones may be involved in mediating some of the actions of the hormones and their analogues, such as are known to involve more long-term intracellular processes.

Receptors do not appear to directly alter or metabolize the agonists or antagonists with which they bind. Dissociation can usually occur without permanent change in either component. Whether or not there is an intermediate structure linking the receptor and enzymes, such as adenylate cyclase, is not clear, although several models have been proposed (Figure 15). It is, however, possible to isolate membrane fragments containing the receptor with its attached adenylate cyclase, which can be activated by hormones, and their analogues, with the resulting formation of cyclic AMP. Solubilized membrane receptors, however, appear to be separated from the enzyme, as this response cannot in those cases be elicited by the hormone. Such preparations, however, still retain their abilities to interact specifically with the hormones.

An excellent description of the methods used to identify and study hormone receptors is provided in a laboratory methods manual prepared by Schrader and O'Malley (1978). The more classical pharmacological methods for analyzing the nature of the interactions of drugs and receptors from their dose–response relationships, and the analysis of the interactions of radioactively labelled drugs and their receptors, have been described by Furchgott (1978).

Architecture of a receptor

Diabetes mellitus is the most common endocrine disease, and in the United States it is the third most common cause of death. Although the administration of insulin prolongs life, it does not, at this time, prevent the long-term adverse effects of the disease on the vascular and nervous systems. There has thus been considerable interest in the role and

Figure 15. Models of possible physical relationships between hormone receptors and adenylate cyclase. (a) Single molecule. (b) Physical coupling models: (i) stable association tandem or triplet schemes; (ii) mobile receptor hypothesis. (c) Indirect interaction models. A variety of drugs (agonists and antagonists) may also interact with the hormone receptor. (From Greaves, 1977)

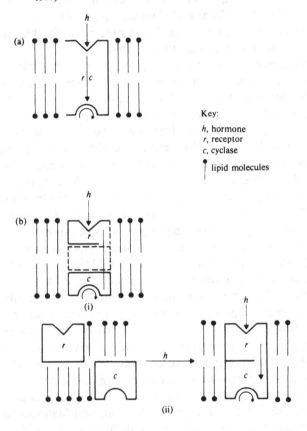

Key:

h, hormone
r, receptor
c, cyclase

| lipid molecules

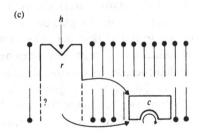

actions of insulin in the body, including the functioning of its receptors, and there is probably more information about the insulin receptor than any other such molecular component of cells (see Cuatrecasas et al., 1975; Roth et al., 1975; Hollenberg and Cuatrecasas, 1978).

The physicochemical nature and behavior of receptors may be unraveled as a result of several types of observations.

First, indirect inferences based on the study of the structure–activity relationships of drugs and natural excitants are often used to create models of what a receptor may look like. Receptors and drugs are thought to combine in a manner that reflects the complementarity of their chemical groups, shape, electrical charges, and clouds of electrons. One is thought to be a type of mirror image of the other. Thus, the nature of the receptor is sometimes inferred from knowledge about the conformation of the drug with which it can combine. An example is shown in Figure 16, which incorporates information about electrical charge, van der Waals forces associated with the aromatic ring, and a bulky projection from the piperidine ring to give a three-point attachment of morphine to its receptor. Additional steric embellishments, often added to such models of receptors, are sculptured ridges, tunnels, and grooves, which will accommodate channels, protrusions, and ridges on the drug. Other properties such as negative-cooperativity behavior in binding with drugs or hormones may be taken to infer a grouping or clustering of receptors. The importance of ions such as Na^+, Ca^{2+}, and Mg^{2+} for drug–receptor interactions may provide information about the possible importance of electrical charges on the receptor and its natural rigidity and ability to change its shape.

Second, more direct observations can now be made on the receptor with the aid of modern biochemical, immunological, and histological techniques. Receptors in tissues can now, with the aid of radioimmunoassay procedures, be counted, and their relative preferences for different molecules compared. Parts of cells, such as the plasma membrane, cytoplasm, and nucleus, can be separated so that the receptors they contain can be prepared in a more concentrated form. They can be further purified using centrifugation techniques, as in sucrose density gradients, and some have even, often with the aid of detergents, been solubilized. It is thus possible in many instances to estimate the size of receptors and determine their chemical constitution. Further information about their chemical makeup can also be derived, either in intact cells or in enriched preparations, from studies of the actions of enzymes and chemicals with known specific actions, such as SH-reactive compounds, like *p*-chloromercuriphenyl sulfonic acid (PCMPS), and plant lectins (e.g., concanavalin A), which interact with carbohydrate moieties. The actions of such enzymes and reagents on the binding of drugs, or the responses to them, may be taken to infer the presence and importance of certain constituents of the receptors. Antibodies can also be prepared to purified receptors and can be used to aid their identification. A number of fluorescent dyes are available that make it possible to label receptors so they can be directly observed and photographed, even in living cells.

Figure 16. Diagrammatic three-dimensional representation of the morphine receptor based on the structure–activity relationships of the drug. The diagram represents the lower surface of the drug and the upper surface of the receptor, that is, complementary surfaces in front (➡), behind (- - -), and in the plane (—), of the paper. Three essential sites of the receptor are depicted: (1) a flat surface allowing for the binding with the aromatic ring through van der Waals–type forces; (2) an anionic site that associates with the positive charge, associated with the N, in the center of the drug; and (3) a cavity oriented to sites 1 and 2 to accommodate the projecting portion —CH_2—CH_2 of the piperidine ring (in front of the plane of the paper). (From Beckett and Casy, 1954, *J. Pharm. Pharmacol.*, with permission)

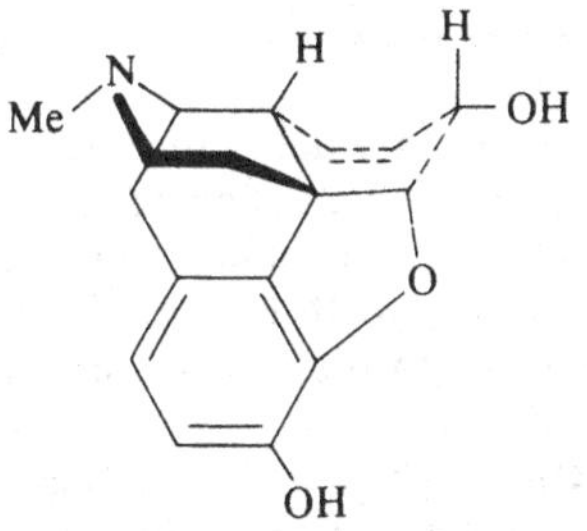

(−)-Morphine

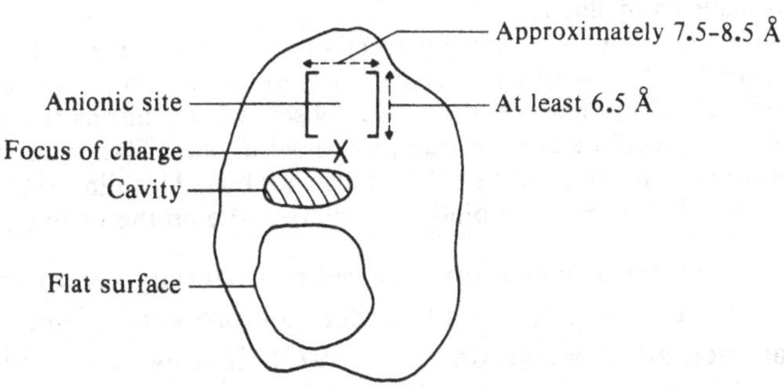

Approximately 7.5–8.5 Å

Anionic site

At least 6.5 Å

Focus of charge

Cavity

Flat surface

Receptor surface

Such studies have provided a wealth of information about the nature and properties of the insulin receptor:

1. It is a glycoprotein with a molecular weight of about 300,000 daltons.
2. Incubation with lipolytic enzymes shows that it is partially buried in the cell membranes and faces in an outward direction. Its activity can be destroyed by trypsin.
3. Insulin combines with its receptor reversibly and is not directly changed or destroyed following such a combination. The dissociation constant, K_D, is about 10^{-10}M.
4. The response to the insulin appears to be maximal when only about 5 percent of the receptors are occupied. This phenomenon has been described in many pharmacological preparations and appears to reflect a reserve of spare receptors.
5. There is an interaction between the receptors so that dissociation of the hormone from them is enhanced as their occupation increases (at physiological levels where 1 to 5 percent are normally occupied). The equilibrium constant K_D increases with the occupancy of the receptors, a phenomenon known as negative cooperativity (DeMeyts et al., 1976). This effect may reflect a change in the nature of the receptor or its site in the membrane.
6. The distribution of the receptors in the cell may be influenced by the microfilament system, as binding can be reduced by cytochalasin A, B, and D.
7. The insulin receptors can interact with other types of molecules including the plant lectin protein concanavalin A and wheat germ agglutin, and other peptides, including somatomedins, epidermal growth factor, and nerve growth factor. These substances can displace ^{125}I-insulin in proportion to their endogenous insulin-like activity.
8. The continued presence of high concentration of insulin reduces (= "down regulation") the number of insulin receptors. This phenomenon could reflect a regulatory mechanism for controlling the effects of insulin, and it may be involved in the onset of certain types of diabetes mellitus.
9. Antibodies to purified insulin receptors have been prepared. It is interesting that they not only can bind to the receptors but can also elicit an insulin-like response. This observation confirms that such isolated receptors are the true physiological ones. The antibodies to insulin receptors, however, do not displace bound insulin, so that each agonist thus appears to bind to a different site on the receptor.

The identification of ^{125}I-insulin, by radioautography, on the plasma membrane of liver cells appears to reflect the presence of specific receptors at such sites (Bergeron et al., 1977). However, using similar methods it has been shown that following a period of incubation the labelled insulin is translocated, probably along with its receptor, into a region inside the cell periphery (Gorden et al., 1978). Fluorescent analogues of insulin have also been prepared which have allowed direct observation of the movements of the polypeptide molecule in living fibroblast cells (Schlessinger et al., 1978). Initially the hormone was seen to be associated with the plasma membrane, in which it could move in a lateral plane. Subsequently, after about 30 minutes, it became immobile and appeared in endocytotic vesicles in the cell cytoplasm.

It is possible that quantitative and qualitative differences in insulin receptors could result in certain forms of diabetes mellitus.

Nature of the receptor response to a drug

It appears that receptors usually undergo a conformation change as a result of their interaction with a drug that acts as an agonist. This effect can be likened to that of the interaction of a ligand for the allosteric site on an allosteric protein or enzyme (see, e.g., Changeux et al., 1967; Karlin, 1967; Rang, 1971; Thron, 1973). However, it is doubtful, despite earlier speculation, that the receptor always constitutes a permanent component of an enzyme or is an enzyme per se. The receptor-drug complex sooner or later may interact with an enzymic system and alter its activity, but it has been shown in many instances to be a separate dissociable entity. A conformational change in the receptor may have several effects, including its subsequent dissociation into subunits, promotion of movement from the cytoplasm to the nucleus, a lateral migration within the plasma membrane, or even transfer from the latter into the cytoplasm. The change may also promote an association of the receptor with enzymes, such as in the chromatin or with membrane adenylate cyclase (see Chapter 10). In the instance of "fixed" receptors which may be a part (even a regulatory allosteric site) of an enzyme, the binding of the drug may have a more direct, allosteric-like effect on its conformation and hence change its activity.

Control of receptor function

There appears to be a continual process of degradation and renewal ("turnover") of many receptors. It is thus not surprising to observe that their numbers may vary in response to drugs and hormones, and in disease. Such changes may account for variations in the sensitivity of a target tissue to a drug. A deficiency of receptors for insulin, and androgenic steroids, has been observed in certain diseases. This can be genetic or reflect environmental changes. Thus, high circulating levels of insulin have been observed to bring about a decline in the number of their own, but not other types of receptors. Hormones may control the synthesis of the heterologous receptors; for instance, estrogens can stimulate the formation of progesterone receptors and α-adrenergic receptors. Some drugs can inhibit the formation of receptors; the antiestrogen tamoxifen thus appears to block synthesis of estrogen receptors. The formation of new hormone receptors involves protein synthesis and can be inhibited by actinomycin D or puromycin.

The interaction between a hormone (and possibly also drugs) and its receptor may be self-regulating as a result of changes in the affinity of the receptor. This phenomenon has been observed with a number of hormones including insulin. When the concentration of the hormone is raised, its binding to the receptors declines and the K_D increases. This

Figure 17. A model to describe the activation and inactivation of β-adrenergic receptors in the presence of β-adrenergic agonists such as isoproterenol. "Rapid" activation responses occur in seconds, whereas subsequent desensitization and reactivation are "slow" and take minutes. For details see text. (From Lefkowitz, 1976. Reprinted by permission from *The New England Journal of Medicine* 295:327)

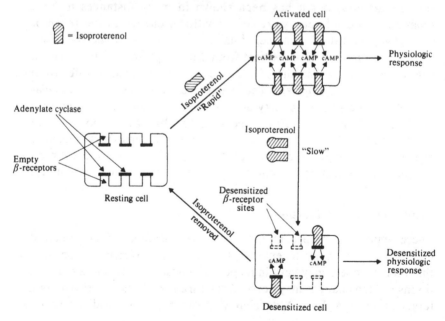

process, mentioned earlier in this chapter (under "Architecture of a receptor"), is called negative cooperativity. From the practical, functional standpoint it is best to consider the converse of this situation, in which the sensitivity of the receptors is greatest when the concentration of a hormone is low. This phenomenon also suggests that certain types of receptors may interact with each other; they are probably closely associated in "clusters" on the cell membrane.

The prolonged exposure of β-adrenergic receptors to the β-adrenergic agonist isoproterenol results in a progressive decline in the response, a production of cyclic AMP. This "desensitization" has been observed in frog erythrocyte membranes and a line of mouse lymphoma cells. These preparations can still, however, respond to other types of agonists, such as prostaglandins and cholera toxin. The effect is not seen when the preparation is exposed to a β-adrenergic antagonist. The change in sensitivity is accompanied by a loss of β-adrenergic receptors, which, once the agonist is removed, are gradually restored. A model to describe and account for these effects is shown in Figure 17. (The subject of hormonal regulation of receptors has been reviewed in detail by Catt et al., 1979.)

9
Relationship of chemical structure to biological activity

Individual chemical compounds and drugs can elicit particular, and often unique, biological responses. Effects may be confined to the substance involved, or to a group of substances, and be determined by a variety of physicochemical properties of the active compound. The properties of such a reactive molecule that influence its ability to have an effect include its shape, size, electrical charge, distribution of electrons, chemically reactive groups, and intramolecular distances between parts of the molecule that are involved in its interaction with its receptor.

Ideally a complete knowledge and understanding of the importance of such chemical and structural factors, with respect to each type of drug–receptor interaction, could provide a rational basis for the design of drugs with specified properties. The availability of sophisticated computers makes such a prospect more likely (see Gund et al., 1980), but such mathematical predictions or quantitative structure–activity relationships (QSAR) are not yet generally available as a predictive tool. The random screening of compounds for biological activity is time-consuming and expensive, but it is still carried out. However, application of knowledge, limited as it may be, of the relationship of chemical structure to a biological activity can narrow the field of search, though it is still quite empirical. This guided approach usually follows the recognition of some structural correlate to the molecule's biological activity in a particular group of drugs. It is often possible in such situations to modify the chemical structure in order to increase or decrease the potency of the drug, make an antagonist to it, or modify the spectrum of its actions, side effects, and toxicity. In many, but not all, instances it is possible to make reasonably accurate predictions as to the effect that a certain chemical change may have on the activity of the molecule. The information that is available, however, is usually gained initially using an empirical approach.

72

The effects of such structural changes on a drug's actions may be direct or indirect.

Direct effects influence the molecule's ability to combine with its receptor and/or initiate a response. The two parts of the molecule that are considered to confer such properties are called (1) the binding site, address sequence, or recognon; and (2) the active site, message sequence, catalytic site, or acton. Recognition of the properties of each such part of the molecule can be of considerable help in drug design. Unfortunately, however, these two parts of the molecule may not be entirely separate or independent of each other, and often one cannot be changed without influencing the other. This problem is not surprising when one considers the importance of the shape of a molecule for both its affinity and its intrinsic activity and the inherent difficulties in changing the constitution of one part of the molecule without altering its overall three-dimensional configuration.

Indirect effects, not related to the drug–receptor interaction, of changes in a drug's structure on its biological activity, are also of considerable practical importance in designing drugs. Such changes may influence a drug's absorption from the site of administration, its distribution in the body (e.g., accumulation in fat or ability to cross the blood–brain barrier), its binding to plasma proteins, its metabolism, as a result of the action of enzymes, and its excretion in the urine and bile.

Certain general chemical characters that influence such properties of drugs, including their lipid solubility and electrical charge, can usually be readily recognized and are associated with specific chemical moieties present in the molecule. However, a more complete understanding depends on the unraveling of the three-dimensional shape of the molecule, including the direction and alignment of the chemical groups and side chains about its surfaces, which may promote or hinder its activities. Such studies are usually made using physical techniques such as X-ray crystallography and nuclear magnetic resonance (NMR) spectroscopy.

As just described, the biological activity of a chemical compound, whether a drug or a natural excitant, is related to the physical and chemical reactivities of the chemical moieties it contains, as well as its three-dimensional shape. Peptides are important natural compounds that may act as hormones and neurotransmitters, and, although they are quite complex, they can be readily synthesized, so that one constituent amino acid can be substituted for another. The three-dimensional configurations of a number of such natural compounds investigated in this way were those hormones that are secreted by the neu-rohypophysis, a lobe of the pituitary gland. These compounds are nonapeptides, consisting of a ring of six amino acids and an acyclic side chain containing three more (Figure 18). The natural hormones in man are antidiuretic hormone (ADH, also called vasopressin) and oxytocin. ADH reduces urine flow by acting on the kidney and in high doses also constricts blood vessels (pressor effect), including the coronaries in the heart. Oxytocin can contract the uterus during parturition and also promotes the release of milk from the mammary gland (galactobolic effect). There is little (< 5 percent) crossover in these actions of the two peptide hormones even though they only differ from each other by two amino acid substitutions, at the 3- and 8-positions (Figure 18).

More than 300 structural variants, or analogues, based on these two hormones have been made in the laboratory, and the spectra of their biological activities have been examined. One of the first such analogues to be made was a combination of the side chain of ADH (or vasopressin) and the ring section on oxytocin. (Hence it was called vasotocin.) This peptide was found to possess activity characteristic of both of its parent molecules; it had substantial antidiuretic, pressor, oxytocic, and galactobolic effects. (It is interesting that this was origi-nally a synthetic peptide but was subsequently found to be present in many nonmammalian vertebrates.) Such a relatively clear illustration of chemical structure as related to biological activity is, however, quite rare among such peptides. The precise reason for the association of a particular part of the molecule to a certain biological action is also usually obscure. Generally such relationships are only found by empir-ical observation, though catalogs of such information can be exceed-ingly useful when one is attempting to design new compounds.

Desmopressin is an analogue of ADH that was recently introduced into clinical practice for reducing urine flow in diabetes insipidus. Natural ADH can be used to replace the deficient hormone, but its action is quite short-lived, about 3 to 4 hours in duration. Removal of the amino group from the cystine in position 1 prolongs the action of such peptides, as this change hinders the activity of aminopeptidases, which destroy ADH in the body. It has also been observed that when D-arginine is used to replace the natural L-arginine at the 8-position in ADH, then both the antidiuretic and pressor activities of the molecule decline. However, the latter activity is reduced much more so that the molecule has an antidiuretic/pressor activity ratio of 28 : 1. The precise reason for this change in relative activity is uncertain, but it may reflect

Figure 18. Primary structures of oxytocin and vasopressin showing the amino acid side chains. These hormones consist of a 20-membered ring which is closed by a disulfide bridge between the two half-cystines at positions 1 and 6, and a peptide side chain containing three amino acids. The two hormones differ by the presence of two amino acids at positions 3 and 8. (From Jard and Bockaert, 1975)

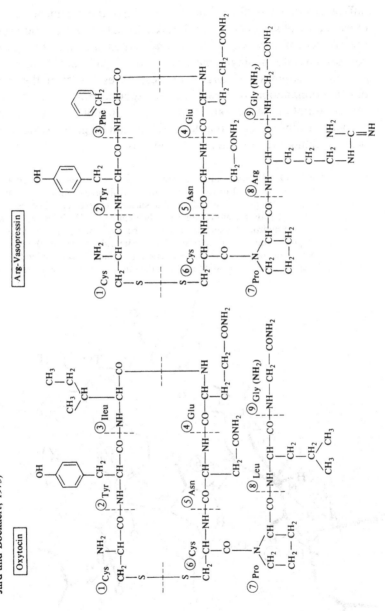

differences in the local rates of inactivation of the peptide in the vicinity of each type of its receptor, or differences between the antidiuretic and pressor receptor–peptide interactions. When the two changes are incorporated into a single molecule, so as to make 1-deamino-8-D-arginine vasopressin (DDAVP or desmopressin), then the molecule has a combination of desirable therapeutic effects: It has a prolonged duration of action, up to about 20 hours, and it has little vasoconstrictor effect so that large doses can be given without the risk of contracting the coronary blood vessels.

Figure 19. (a) Urry-Walter "cooperative model," showing the proposed tertiary structure of oxytocin in its biologically active form in aqueous solution. One plane, the hydrophobic surface, is essentially featureless except for the protruding disulfide bond and the peptide N—H of glutamine. The other side, the hydrophilic surface, involves the Tyr^2, Asn^5, Gln^4, and the linear tripeptide sequence of oxytocin. The model utilizes each of the constituent amino acids to its greatest effectiveness to achieve formation and intramolecular stabilization of the backbone to which the side chains of Cys^1,

(a)

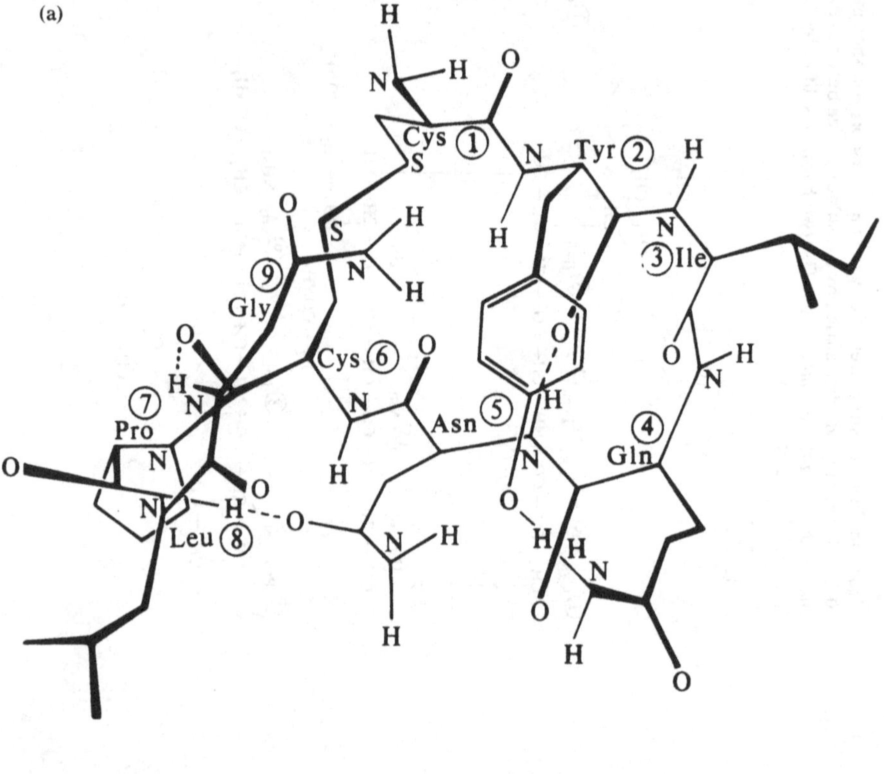

A rational approach to the design of a drug must also depend on a knowledge of its three-dimensional structure, which will usually, of necessity, incorporate empirically derived information about the importance of the various chemical groups that it contains. Thus, although it may be known that a certain amide, carbonyl, alkyl, or guanidinium group may be important for biological activity, knowledge of the group's position and spatial alignment is also vital. For instance, it may become apparent that such a group is important to maintain the shape of the backbone of the molecule, or it may need to have a special

Caption to Fig. 19 (*cont.*)
Cys[6], Tyr[2], and Asn[5] contribute. The side chains of Ile[3], Gln[4], Pro[7], and Leu[8] are considered to be free to engage in intermolecular interactions, while having a limited effect on the conformation of the peptide backbone, with the exception of the corner residue Pro, in view of its relative rigidity. (From Walter, 1977) (b) Proposed tertiary structure of lysine-vasopressin in aqueous solution. The backbone structure also applies to arginine-vasopressin. (From Walter et al., 1977)

alignment in relation to a particular surface of the molecule. In 1971, Urry and Walter, largely on the basis of NMR spectroscopy studies, provided a three-dimensional model for the structure of oxytocin (Figure 19a). They later extended this to ADH (Figure 19b). The ring section of oxytocin has a right-handed helical twist, or β-turn, involving the -Tyr-Ile-Gln-Asn (positions 2 to 5 in the molecule) sequence of amino acids. The disulfide bond provided by the two half-cystines is of basic importance in maintaining the ring structure, but the configuration is also stabilized by intramolecular hydrogen bonds, the most notable being that between the carbonyl (C=O) of the 2-tyrosine and the amide (NH) of the 5-asparagine. The latter amino acid appears to play a pivotal role in maintaining the structure of these peptides, and even its slight modification always results in drastic decreases in biological activity. Its importance appears to lie largely in its role in helping to maintain the shape of the backbone of the molecule. Another such intramolecular stabilizing hydrogen bond in oxytocin exists between the amide on the 9-glycine and the carbonyl on the 6-half-cystine. Superimposed on this basic backbone structure are the various amino acid side-chain groups, which provide the intermolecular bonds necessary for the appropriate binding of the excitant to its receptor. In oxytocin these moieties include the side chains supplied by the 3-isoleucine, 4-glutamine, 7-proline, and 8-leucine substituents. In ADH the 3-phenylalanine and the 8-arginine substituents are important.

Oxytocin and vasopressin appear to have two major surfaces, a hydrophobic one, which is fairly featureless except for the disulfide group and the amide of glutamine, and a hydrophilic surface, from which the other groups protrude and are free to engage in intermolecular interactions such as are necessary to bind the molecule to its receptor. Other side chains may, however, be important for the expression of the peptide's intrinsic activity. These include the carboxamide of the 5-asparagine, the aromatic ring of the 2-tyrosine in oxytocin, and the basic guanidinium side chain of the 8-arginine in antidiuretic hormone. Eventually it is hoped that the use of this type of information about the precise conformation of such molecules will allow a more accurate prediction of their biological activity and allow for their design in a more rational, less empiric, manner.

10

Roles of the cell membrane in responses to drugs

The cell membrane (see Figure 20) always plays a role in the actions of drugs, and sometimes is the ultimate site of their response. Cells are enveloped by the plasma membrane, which can restrict and regulate the movements of molecules, including drugs, between their internal contents and the external bathing solutions. This membrane can also receive, and respond to, signals from the inside and outside of the cell. It thus can act as a communications network and transmit external messages, which initiate responses inside the cell, and it can also act as an effector mechanism for the cell.

Cell membranes are composed mostly of lipids, but they also contain proteins, carbohydrates, and some minerals, notably calcium. These components are arranged in an orderly manner. The precise composition of the membrane may, however, differ in various types of tissues and organs. The characteristic architecture and components of cell membranes appear to be related to the special functions of each type of cell. Thus, although a nerve (or muscle) cell membrane can, as in most cells, maintain a difference in electrical charge between its two surfaces, this electrical potential difference (PD) can be made to change rapidly so that a flow of current, constituting a nerve impulse, flows across its surface. The facility to do this is due to the presence of special "channels" through which Na and K ions can move from one side of the membrane to the other. Other types of cells, such as those lining the gut and in the liver, have membranes that are specialized to take up certain nutrients and perform certain other functions, thus also offering potential sites for the actions of drugs. The plasma membrane is also the site where many receptors for drugs and hormones, especially the peptides, are present. (Receptors were discussed in Chapter 8; see especially under "Nature of receptors" and "Architecture of a receptor.") Such receptors usually appear to be glycoproteins.

Most drugs that enter, and leave, cells cross the plasma membrane by the process of diffusion. Although water-soluble substances may pass through aqueous channels, these channels make up only a small proportion of the total surface area of the cell, and they will not accommodate molecules with a molecular weight larger than 100 to 150 daltons. Most drugs are larger than this. Because cell membranes are composed mainly of lipids, it is not surprising to observe that drugs that are readily soluble in oil diffuse across the plasma membrane more readily than water-soluble drugs. The relative solubility of a compound in oil as compared to water is called its *partition coefficient*. Measurement of the partition coefficient can be made using an olive oil/water mixture or a lipid solvent, such as chloroform/water, the pH being standardized (usually 7.4). Such partition coefficients of drugs have been found to predict, with reasonable accuracy, the relative rates at which different drugs may cross cell membranes, a high partition coefficient indicating a more ready access. (A value greater than 0.01, for oil/water, is considered to suggest a significant ability to cross such a membrane.) The ability to leave a water phase and enter a lipid phase, such as the cell membrane, will ultimately depend on the chemical structure of the compound. It will be opposed by the presence of polar,

Figure 20. Diagrammatic model of the plasma membrane depicting its two enveloping, lipid monolayers and the proteins and carbohydrates that float in this matrix. Neither the lipids, proteins, nor their attached carbohydrate moieties are uniform in different types of cells, but they are made up of different molecular components. The proteins and glycoproteins contribute various functions, including receptors for hormones (and drugs), channels through which polar molecules, such as ions, can pass, and enzymes that mediate some communicative events between the inside and outside of the cell. (From Lodish and Rothman, 1979. Copyright 1979 by *Scientific American*, Inc. All rights reserved)

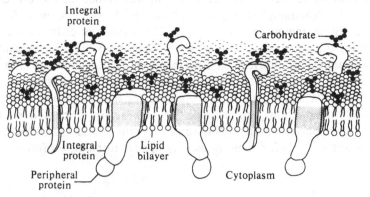

or hydrophilic, groups in the molecule; for example, amino ($-NH_2$), hydroxyl ($-OH$), and carboxyl ($-COOH$) moieties, which tend to form hydrogen bonds with water. On the other hand, it will be facilitated by methyl groups and benzene rings, which enhance solubility in lipids. Cationic and anionic charges strongly oppose entry into lipids, owing to their strong associations with water molecules. The overall lipid solubility of a drug will depend on the balance of such forces, but the presence of ionized groups will tend to override all else so that the molecule will, for practical purposes, then be lipid-insoluble.

An example of the relationship of the actions of drugs to the partition coefficient is provided by different barbiturate drugs. *Thiopental* has a chloroform/water partition coefficient of about 100, and so is highly soluble in lipids. This drug is used for general anesthesia, and when given by intravenous infusion it has a rapid onset of action, readily crossing the blood–brain barrier. When the infusion is stopped, however, its effects rapidly subside, principally because of a redistribution of the drug within the body. Thus, its lipid solubility also allows it to enter many other tissues so that it becomes diluted. The relatively high lipid solubility of thiopental mainly reflects the presence of the $C=S$ moiety. *Phenobarbital* is a sedative-hypnotic that lacks such a chemical group, and it has a chloroform/water partition coefficient of about 2. Although this value is low compared to that of thiopental, it is still sufficient to assure, for practical use, the absorption of the drug after oral administration, and an ability to cross the blood–brain barrier, where it exerts its effects. Its action is, however, slower in onset and more prolonged than that of thiopental. In addition, 25 to 50 percent of the phenobarbital is excreted in the urine, whereas virtually no thiopental is eliminated in this manner. (The latter is mainly degraded in the liver.) Such differences in the manner of elimination of the two drugs also partly reflect their respective abilities to cross cell membranes; any thiopental that is filtered at the glomerulus would be expected to be reabsorbed much more readily than the phenobarbital. Thiopental is also more readily metabolized. At the extreme of the spectrum of lipid solubility is the ganglionic blocking drug *hexamethonium*. Its chloroform/water partition coefficient is about zero, reflecting the presence of two cationic quaternary ammonium groups on the molecule. This drug was an early prototype for the treatment of hypertension; however, it is not absorbed appreciably across the gastrointestinal tract, and so must be injected. It is readily excreted, unchanged, in the urine so that it also has to be administered frequently. For these, and other, reasons it is clearly not an ideal antihypertensive drug. A potential advantage, however, is that it cannot enter the brain. The abilities of drugs to cross cell membranes clearly can have important consequences with respect to their therapeutic actions.

Most drugs are relatively large molecules and are often electrolytes, so that they form salts. Because they are usually weak acids and bases, their degree of dissociation, or ionization, is profoundly influenced by the pH of the solution in which they are present. Examples of weak acids include phenobarbital, aspirin, and phenylbutazone, which, when dissociated, are anions. Weak bases, in which the drug is a cation, include amphetamines, procainamide, and nortriptylene. The pH of the different body fluids may vary considerably; the plasma and interstitial fluids are at about pH 7.4, but the pH of gastric juices is between 1 and 3, whereas the pH of fluids of the intestinal tract and the urine varies between about 5 and 8. Thus the degree of ionization of such drugs and therefore their propensity to cross cell membranes, which only occurs appreciably in their nonionized, or electrically neutral form, may differ considerably within the body.

The ability of a particular drug to become ionized under specific conditions is related to its dissociation or ionization constant, or K_a. For a weak acid, the K_a can be quite low, for instance, 10^{-11}. A more convenient way of expressing such a value is to take its negative logarithm, called its pK_a, which in this example would be 11. The pK_a is equal to the pH when 50 percent of the drug is ionized.

If the pK_a of the drug and the pH of the solution in which it is present are known, it is then possible to calculate the percent of the drug that is nonionized and so potentially able to cross a cell membrane. The relative concentrations of a drug on two sides of a membrane at equilibrium can also be estimated. Whether such a process will actually occur or not, will, however, depend on the innate lipid solubility of the particular neutral molecule; a lack of ionization does *not* assure that the drug can actually cross a lipid membrane.

To calculate the ratio of the nonionized to the ionized concentrations of a drug that is a weak acid, the mass action law is applied as follows:

$$AH \underset{\text{(weak acid)}}{} \rightleftharpoons \underset{\text{(anion)}}{A^-} + \underset{\text{(cation)}}{H^+}$$

$$\underset{\substack{\text{(dissociation} \\ \text{constant or} \\ \text{ionization} \\ \text{constant)}}}{K_a} = \frac{[A^-][H^+]}{[AH]} \tag{1}$$

As described above, it is convenient to convert the K_a to a whole number by taking its negative logarithm, which is its pK_a:

$$pK_a = -\log_{10} K_a$$

The higher the pK_a, the weaker the acid. For the purpose of the calculations, and to relate the K_a to the hydrogen ion concentration (the pH), it is convenient to convert equation (1) into logarithmic form. Hence:

$$\log K_a = \log[H^+] + \log \frac{[A^-]}{[AH]} \tag{2}$$

Rearranging:

$$-\log[H^+] = -\log K_a + \log \frac{[A^-]}{[AH]} \tag{3}$$

$$-\log[H^+] = pH \quad \text{and} \quad -\log K_a = pK_a$$

Hence we can substitute these terms:

$$pH - pK_a = \log \frac{[A^-]}{[AH]} \tag{4}$$

(This is the *Henderson-Hasselbach equation*.)
Or:

$$pH - pK_a = \log \frac{[\text{ionized acid}]}{[\text{nonionized acid}]} \tag{5}$$

In a more general form:

$$pH - pK_a = \log \frac{[\text{proton acceptor}]}{[\text{proton donor}]} \tag{6}$$

The use of this general equation (6) allows us to make a similar calculation of the dissociation of a weak base:

$$\underset{\substack{\text{(weak base or} \\ \text{proton donor)}}}{BH^+} \rightleftharpoons \underset{\substack{\text{(proton} \\ \text{acceptor)}}}{B} + H^+$$

$$\underset{\substack{\text{(for a weak} \\ \text{base)}}}{K_a} = \frac{[H^+][B]}{[BH^+]}$$

Then, as in equations (3) and (4):

$$pH - pK_a = \log \frac{[B]}{[BH^+]} \tag{7}$$

or, as also derived from equation (6):

$$pH - pK_a = \log \frac{[\text{nonionized base}]}{[\text{ionized base}]} \tag{8}$$

The proteins in the plasma membrane provide channels through which hydrophilic and electrically charged molecules, including some drugs, can pass. The Na-channel is one of these membrane proteins. Many drugs can act directly, or indirectly via neurotransmitters, to initiate or hinder changes in the electrical polarization of the membranes of nerve and muscle cells. The drug effects appear to involve changes in the numbers and properties of such ion channels, which can be quite selective for certain ions. For instance, they may discriminate between Na^+, K^+, and Ca^{2+}. An especially interesting example of such an effect is that of the paralytic poison *tetrodotoxin,* which was first identified as a result of observing the fatal effects of eating poorly fileted puffer fish. The skin of certain newts and frogs, and the poison glands of some octopuses, also contain this very toxic chemical. Tetrodotoxin can specifically block Na-channels in the plasma membranes of nerve and some muscle cells and so prevents the initiation and spread of excitation currents, producing a paralysis. *Local anesthetic drugs* also act in this general manner, by blockading ion channels. Other types of cells also possess ion channels, but they may have somewhat different properties. The process of the reabsorption of salts from the renal glomerular filtrate involves the movement of Na^+ across the renal tubular cells. The Na-channels in these cells can be blocked by the diuretic drugs *amiloride* and *triampterine* (but not by tetrodotoxin) so that salt excretion in the urine increases.

The permeability of cells to ions is continually changing, either for brief periods, as when a nerve or muscle membrane is being depolarized, or for longer periods, as when Na is being reabsorbed across the wall of the distal renal tubule. These processes may involve the creation of new ion channels or the opening and closing of those that are a regular part of the membrane's architecture. Some hormones, neurotransmitters, and drugs may influence such events. The steroid hormone *aldosterone* promotes the reabsorption of Na from the urine, which it appears to do by initiating the formation of new Na-channels. The response can be blocked, though for practical purposes only in vitro, by inhibitors of protein synthesis. The diuretic drug *spironolactone* can also, however, prevent this response in vivo, but it does so by acting as a competitive antagonist of the hormone at its receptor sites.

Normally after a nerve or muscle cell has been depolarized, a process that reflects an opening of Na-channels, the membrane becomes repolarized owing to a closure or "inactivation" of these channels. Some drugs can prevent this latter process, and so promote a longer period of depolarization. The insecticide DDT can have such an effect, though it is not normally encountered in vivo. The veratrum alkaloids are drugs that are obtained from the rhizome of a lily (*Veratrum album*) and have had a place in folk medicine for a long time; some of the components of these plant extracts, including *veratridine,* can also prevent the inactivation of Na-channels. The latter drug has been used to lower blood pressure in hypertensive disease. Its effect is due largely to its action on baroreceptors in the carotid sinus, so that the reflex decline in blood pressure that these sites mediate is triggered at a lower basal blood pressure than usual. It appears that because there are more open Na-channels, the effector mechanism falsely perceives a higher blood pressure and thus overreacts. This drug can apparently exert such effects at other sites in the body, and this behavior may account for its side effects, especially nausea and vomiting, which are so troublesome that the drug is not considered useful today. (It, however, appears to have retained a place in veterinary medicine where it can be used to induce vomiting in pigs.)

A number of substances have been identified that can increase the permeability of cell membranes to polar molecules, often to specific ions such as Na^+, K^+, and Ca^{2+}. Such changes can perturb the activities of cells, often mimicking biological responses such as contracting a muscle, depolarizing a nerve, or making an exocrine or endocrine gland secrete its products. Few of these types of compounds have at this time proved to be therapeutically useful as drugs, principally because of their widespread actions in the body. They are, however, of considerable theoretical interest, not only as toxins and venoms, but as tools for research into the activities of cells. The prototypes of such compounds have usually originated as an extract or secretion of some other organism, either animal or microorganism. These sources include spiders, and exotic species of frogs and snakes. The substances appear to function as part of such animals' armamentaria, serving for their protection or as an aid in catching their prey.

Some drugs can enter the plasma membrane, become lodged in the lipid, and so disrupt its normal orderliness and permeability properties, creating aqueous "pores" in it. Amphotericin B is an antibiotic that can combine with sterols; and when it does so with the ergosterol in the cell walls of invading fungal microorganisms, it destroys them. It can, however, also combine with cholesterol, which is present in the membranes of the cells of the animal host; it appears to do this especially readily, or possibly with more devastating effects, in the kidney tubule, and thus can exert serious nephrotoxic actions. The basis for this side effect is also an increase in permeability, the same basic effect that results in its destruction of the fungi.

Valinomycin is a cyclic depsipeptide originally isolated from a microorganism (*Streptomyces fulvissimus*). It can enter lipid membranes and pass from one side of them to the other. Although it can act in this manner because it is lipid-soluble, it also contains a central chamber, or space, into which an ion can be sequestered. Valinomycin thus has a selectivity for alkali metal ions, but has a thousand-fold preference for K^+ as compared to Na^+. It can thus specifically increase the permeability of cell membranes to K^+. A number of carboxylic acid compounds isolated from microorganisms are lipid-soluble and can also carry ions across cell membranes. These compounds include *nigericin*, which carries K, and *monensin*, which has a special affinity for Na. *A23187* transports Ca. Such compounds are called ionophores. Other venoms can, like amphotericin B, make holes or channels in cell membranes and admit ions. Extracts from the skin of a small Colombian frog (*Phyllobates aurotaenia*) are used as an arrow poison for hunting by local Indians. The active principal is a steroidal alkaloid (Albuquerque et al., 1971), which has been called *batrachotoxin*. This poison increases the permeability of nerve and muscle cell membranes to Na^+. The effect is irreversible, but it is interesting that the holes can be blocked with tetrodotoxin. *Crotamine*, a peptide that is present in the venom of a South American rattlesnake, also increases the permeability of cell membranes to Na. The *venom of the black widow spider* contains a number of toxic proteins, which act on the end plate of the neuromuscular junction. One of these substances has been shown to increase permeability of a cultured cell line of neurosecretory cells to Ca^{2+} so that they then release their stored catecholamines (Grasso et al., 1980).

Some membrane proteins function as enzymes, and they can also be influenced by drugs. Sodium ions can be extruded from cells, across their plasma membranes. This process occurs against an electrochemical gradient, and requires the expenditure of energy by the cell. Such mechanisms are called active transport. One of the main events in active Na transport, which involves the breakdown of ATP, is mediated by Na-K activated ATPase, which is present in the cell membrane. This enzyme can be specifically inhibited by the digitalis cardiac glycosides, such as digoxin. These drugs are used therapeutically to increase the force of contraction of heart muscle in congestive heart failure. However, they have a low ratio of therapeutic safety and often also exert toxic effects on the heart. These adverse responses appear to reflect their interference, via an action on Na-K activated ATPase, with the normal ion regulation of the heart cells. The therapeutic action of the cardiac glycosides may also reflect an action on this membrane enzyme, but this possibility is the subject of controversy.

Adenylate cyclase is another ubiquitous membrane protein that is also an enzyme. The cyclic nucleotide cyclic AMP acts as a second messenger, mediating responses to a number of hormones, neurotransmitters, and drugs. Such responses include the state of contractility of muscle, the secretion of endocrine and exocrine glands, neural communication within the brain, and the control of intermediary, mineral, and water metabolism. Adenylate cyclase promotes the formation of cyclic AMP from ATP. (The relationship of this enzyme to receptors in the plasma membrane was described in Chapter 8, under "Nature of receptors.") Cyclic AMP acts as a mediator by activating a protein kinase in the cell, which in turn phosphorylates, and so can change the configuration of, proteins associated with the responses of the effector organs. Such proteins include those that may influence the permeability of the cell membrane to ions and water. Thus, antidiuretic hormone (ADH) increases the permeability of kidney epithelial cells to water via the hormone's activation of adenylate cyclase. The actions of several neurotransmitters in the brain, including dopamine and norepinephrine, also appear to be mediated by cyclic AMP. In these instances the nucleotide may mediate a change in the permeability of the nerve cells to ions, especially Na. Drugs may mimic or oppose such neurohumoral effects by acting either at the receptor sites associated with the adenylate cyclase or at some other stage of the process, such as by inhibiting the enzyme phosphodiesterase, which inactivates cyclic AMP.

The movements of some drugs across cell membranes may involve active transport. Some notable examples are those drugs that are secreted across the renal tubular epithelium into the glomerular filtrate. They include the thiazide diuretics, phenylbutazone, aspirin, and penicillin. The reuptake of norepinephrine by the terminals of nerve cells also involves the activity of an active pump mechanism in cell membranes. It is, however, not completely specific for this neurotransmitter but can transport a number of other amine compounds, including epinephrine, amphetamines, tricyclic antidepressant drugs (such as imipramine and amitriptyline), and guanethidine. The last is a potent drug used to lower blood pressure in people suffering from hypertension. In order to get to its site of action within the nerve terminal it must be taken up by the membrane "amine pump." If patients being treated for hypertension with guanethidine are subsequently given tricyclic antidepressant drugs, their blood pressure may then rise dramatically. This interaction is due to a competition for sites on the amine pump. Iodide, which is a vital constituent of the thyroid hormone, is taken up by the thyroid gland as a result of the activity of an "anion pump." Some other anions can, however, compete with the iodide, including thiocyanate and perchlorate. Such anions thus have antithydroid effects and have even been used clinically for this action.

Calcium is an important component of cell membranes that can directly and indirectly influence the actions of drugs. This mineral is associated with both the lipid and protein components of the membrane. By influencing surface tension and cross-linkages between molecules it helps to maintain its orderly structure. The Ca concentrations in the cell sap are normally very low, about 10^{-7} M, but following stimulation may rise with a resulting cell response, such as a contraction of a muscle cell or the secretion of a hormone from an endocrine cell. This Ca may be made available from several sites, one of which is the plasma membrane itself. The Ca may also cross the cell membrane through special channels. A number of drugs may act on the cell membrane to influence its Ca metabolism and hence the effector responses of cells.

11
Clinical aspects of the actions of drugs

In its clinical use a drug is intended to have a therapeutic action, but it can also promote toxic reactions and have side effects. The latter can reflect deficiencies in a drug's selectivity and may even occur at the same time or with smaller doses than those that are therapeutically effective. Side effects can also result from excessive doses of drugs, which are then said to be at toxic concentrations and ultimately may even result in death. Such toxic effects are often merely extensions of therapeutic effects. Drug concentrations in the blood provide a convenient way of predicting drug effects. Concentrations can be divided into four general levels: the concentration of the drug that is the *threshold* of the therapeutic response, the *maximal* concentration for a therapeutic effect, the concentration where *toxic* effects may be expected to occur, and the *lethal* concentration.

The difference between the maximally effective therapeutic dose and that at which toxic effects may be expected to occur can be large or relatively small, and depends mainly on the drug. The greater the difference between these two concentrations, the safer the drug is expected to be. This safety factor may be expressed in terms of the *therapeutic index,* which is the ratio of the dose that has a lethal effect (LD) to the dose that is therapeutically effective (ED). Thus, the larger the therapeutic index, the safer the drug. The therapeutic index has various meanings; based on animal experiments, it can be calculated as the ratio of the lethal and effective doses expressed as a percentage of the population that responds. For instance the median effective dose and the lethal dose, for 50 percent of the individuals tested, are, respectively, the LD_{50} and the ED_{50}. The ratio LD_{50}/ED_{50} may be used, but a safer expression of the therapeutic index is LD_1/ED_{99} or $LD_{0.1}/ED_{99.9}$. In man, clinical experience may afford a measure of the toxic dose (TD), and one can use TD_1/ED_{99} as a measure of a drug's safety. It should be recalled, however, that many such measurements are based on animal experiments, and one must be careful about extrapolating such estimates to man. In addition, to complicate the problem, there can be considerable variation between the responses of individuals. These differences can be due to various factors: genetic, environmental, nutritional, disease, and prior treatment with other drugs, which will be described later in this chapter. A note of caution is also necessary when comparing blood concentrations, as what may appear to be therapeutically effective in one individual may sometimes be toxic in another. There is no absolute blood concentration of a drug that can with certainty be stated to be therapeutic or toxic, although such measurements can provide important clues as to the likely situation.

Genetic differences in drug responses

It is a common observation that individuals may exhibit considerable variations in their responses to drugs. In some instances it appears that these differences may exist between groups of people, such as those from different geographic areas. A basic reason for such variation in responses to drugs is the age, size, and diet of the individuals. When the number of people responding to a drug is plotted graphically versus the dose of the drug, a continuous distribution is most often seen, usually appearing as a normal (Gaussian) curve with most individuals clustered around the central 50 percent value. Occasionally, however, the distribution may be multivariate so that the plot contains more than one peak. Isoniazid is used to treat tuberculosis, but there are large differences in the required dose. This variation is reflected in the plasma levels that are achieved following a standard dose and is due to differences in the drug's metabolism (Figure 21). In such a situation, some factor appears to predominate over the more usual causes of differences in drug responses, and this factor may reflect common inherited differences. Such genetic factors may be due to single genes or several genes (multifactorial). The study of such inherited variation in responses to drugs has been dubbed "pharmacogenetics," and was excellently described in a monograph by Kalow (1962). The subject has recently been reviewed by Propping (1978).

There may be several types of immediate causes of such a genetically based difference in drug responses. It may be the result of the presence of abnormal enzymes that are responsible for the inactivation or activation of a drug. It can also involve more general differences in the sensitivity of cells, such as the red blood cell, to drugs, an effect that is also ultimately enzymic. Inherited anatomical differences, such as the depth of the anterior chamber of the eye, may also predispose certain individuals to adverse responses to drugs. In some instances there may be diversity in the characteristics and number of receptors (receptor diseases). Such genetic divergence between individuals may not be apparent (i.e., may be "silent") until they are exposed to a particular drug, or it may have such widespread effects in the body that it is associated with an overt inherited disease.

Abnormal enzymes may result in differences in the levels of a drug in the blood, which, at a certain dosage, may produce either a toxic or a therapeutically ineffective response. A number of drugs depend for their inactivation on a process of acetylation that is carried out in the liver under the influence of N-acetyl transferase. Such drugs include isoniazid, hydralazine (an antihypertensive drug), and procainamide (used to treat cardiac arrythmias). The enzymic reaction can limit the rate of metabolism of such drugs. Individuals have been shown to differ markedly in their ability to carry out this acetylation reaction and are broadly classified as slow and rapid inactivators (or acetylators). In the

Figure 21. Plasma concentration following oral administration of 9.7 mg isoniazid per kilogram body weight in 267 members of 53 white (U.S.A.) families. This drug is used to treat tuberculosis. It can be seen that there are two major peaks in the plasma concentrations of the drug. The distribution reflects genetic differences in the ability to inactivate the drug by the enzymic process of acetylation. The proportions vary in different ethnic groups. Responders are sometimes referred to as "slow" and "fast" acetylators. A number of other drugs are metabolized in this manner, and allowances often have to be made in dosage, so as to assure therapeutic effectiveness and lack of toxicity. (From Clark et al., 1968)

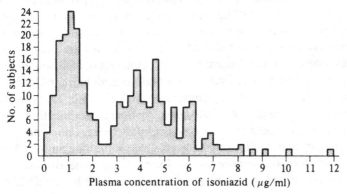

United States 45 percent of white people are rapid inactivators, whereas 55 percent are slow inactivators (see Figure 21). The distribution of these characters is different among the Eskimos, of whom 95 percent are rapid inactivators, and 5 percent are slow inactivators. These enzymic differences are reflected in the blood levels of drugs and can influence their therapeutic and toxic effects. Thus slow inactivators being treated for hypertension with hydralazine may exhibit an enhanced lowering of the blood pressure, compared to rapid inactivators. They also, however, exhibit an increased incidence of a quite common side effect of this drug, a rheumatoid lupus erythematosus-like syndrome.

Primaquine is a drug used to treat malaria. It can, however, in certain individuals cause a hemolytic destruction of red blood cells. This response has been observed to occur more frequently in people from the region of the Mediterranean Sea. This toxic effect of primaquine has a genetic basis and is associated with a deficiency of glucose-6-phosphate dehydrogenase, an enzyme that is necessary to maintain an optimal stability of the red blood cells. The incidence of primaquine sensitivity in Sephardic Jews is about 11 percent, but it is virtually nonexistent in Ashkenazic Jews. It has a high incidence among Greeks, Sardinians, and African blacks, but is absent in Peruvian Indians and Northern Europeans. A number of chemically related drugs, including phenacetin and sulfacetamide, also cause hemolysis in such primaquine-sensitive individuals.

With the recently developed abilities to measure and characterize hormone and drug receptors it has become apparent that genetic differences in responses may also reflect abnormalities in receptors. Several receptor diseases have been characterized that may reflect environmental or genetic variations or even an interaction that involves both of these factors. Diabetes mellitus can sometimes result from a lack of adequate response to endogenous insulin so that more must be administered. There are several examples of receptor diseases involving male steroid sex hormones (androgens), which can result in disorders in sexual differentiation and growth called male pseudohermaphrodism. In some cases the individual may completely lack the ability to respond to endogenous or administered androgens (testicular feminization syndrome), or there may be a relative insensitivity (Reifenstein syndrome or partial androgen insensitivity). These disorders are thought to reflect a lack of receptors for androgens. A form of the bone disease osteomalacia exists that does not respond to treatment with vitamin D or its active metabolite 1,25-(OH)$_2$ vitamin D$_3$. This disease, called vitamin D–resistant rickets, is also thought to be due to an inherited lack of receptors for 1,25-(OH)$_2$vitamin D$_3$.

Tachyphylaxis, tolerance, and dependence

Responses to drugs either in the body (in vivo) or in isolated organs (in vitro) may exhibit a decline following continual periods of stimulation. Thus, larger doses may subsequently be needed to elicit a response than those doses used initially. In a number of cases, especially those involving narcotic drugs which act to depress the central nervous system, this tolerance to the drug action may be accompanied by a physical dependence on its presence. If the drug is withheld, the body may then respond in an adverse hyperexcitable manner that may even result in death. Dependence on a drug may, however, also be more subtle; its effects may be considered to be so pleasant that a psychic craving for it may develop, and its use may then become a habit.

A decline in responses to drugs occurs quite frequently and can be a practical problem, such as in the treatment of hypertension, the maintenance of relief from pain (analgesia), and the use of drugs to promote sleep (hypnotics). The onset of tolerance is generally related to the size of the dose and the duration of its use. It can, however, develop following a single administration of a drug and may persist for many months.

Tachyphylaxis

Tachyphylaxis refers to a rapid decrease in a response to a drug that takes place within minutes of exposure to it. Repeated doses are usually required to elicit such an effect. This type of decline in response is sometimes referred to as *acute tolerance*. Sensitivity will usually return following a period of time when no further doses of the drug are given. Tachyphylaxis commonly occurs under experimental conditions in isolated organ systems, such as pieces of muscle, which are continually stimulated. It is specific to the particular drug used. Tachyphylaxis is also seen experimentally in vivo. Thus, vasopressin (ADH) when injected in large doses, intravenously, into anesthetized rats produces an increase in their blood pressure. However, with frequent repeated doses of this peptide, usually within a few minutes of each other, the response declines. If the doses are sufficiently spaced, at about 30-minute intervals, the effect will not be seen, as sensitivity will return in the meantime. The tachyphylaxis to the vasopressin is quite specific; if epinephrine is injected into such a rat, the response to the latter is unaffected. The mechanism for tachyphylaxis is uncertain, but it is generally thought to involve a temporary depletion of some essential metabolite, a change in the ion content of the tissue, or a change in the properties of the receptor. Tachyphylaxis does not appear to be a common problem in clinical practice, where it is unusual for drugs to be administered repeatedly in such an acute fashion.

Tolerance

Tolerance is a decline in the response to a drug that occurs more gradually than tachyphylaxis. It is seen following the use of a drug over a period of several days or weeks. It can be considered a form of adaptation by the tissue to the presence of a foreign chemical, and is also referred to as *drug resistance*. Following the cessation of use of the drug, tolerance can be quite persistent, and it may still be apparent more than a year later. It is sometimes observed that when tolerance to one drug belonging to a certain chemical group develops, this decline in response is also seen when other drugs of the same group are administered, a phenomenon known as *cross-tolerance*. Tolerance may be the result of a general response of the body, but it is usually confined to an individual tissue. It has, for instance, even been observed in cell cultures in vitro. Tolerance can, however, result from changes in pharmacokinetic factors such as drug absorption, metabolism, binding, and excretion. However, pharmacodynamic changes can occur that more directly influence the effector's response. Thus the hyperactivity of physiological compensatory mechanisms, in the same tissue or at parallel sites, may mediate the decline in sensitivity. There may also be changes in the properties of the receptors for the drug.

Dependence

Physical dependence. Physical dependence is associated with the actions of many narcotic drugs that depress the activity of the central nervous system. The nerve tissues behave as if they have adapted to the presence of the drug, so that their response to it is reduced, and they then are tolerant. If the drug is subsequently withdrawn, however, they then become unstable and respond abnormally. It has been pointed out that physical dependence is the price that is paid for adaptation (or tolerance) to the presence of a drug. The withdrawal of such a drug, or the administration of one of its antagonists, can result in an adverse physical response called the *abstinence syndrome* or *withdrawal illness*. This reaction usually takes the form of an excitation originating in the central nervous system, which may result in such symptoms as nausea, vomiting, sweating, hypopyrexia, insomnia, anxiety, psychotic behavior, and hallucinations. The particular pattern depends on the type of drug involved. Death from cardiovascular collapse may occur.

Drug dependence is a general descriptive term recommended by a committee of the World Health Organization and the United States National Academy of Sciences. It is used to describe the general phenomenon of compulsive drug-seeking behavior whether it involves physical dependence or habituation involving "recreational" drugs. The term addiction has been eschewed for reasons that are not completely clear.

Physical drug dependence occurs in response to the opium group of drugs, such as morphine, heroin, pethidine, and codeine, and probably even to commonly used "mild" analgesics such as pentazocine and propoxyphene (Darvon). Other centrally acting depressant drugs with which physical dependence may occur are the barbiturates, ethanol, and antianxiety drugs, such as diazepam (Valium). Initially such drugs may be used to induce sensations such as elation, euphoria, independence, sedation, and relaxation. Subsequently, however, the desire to avoid the abstinence syndrome may play an essential role in the drive to obtain the drugs.

Psychogenic dependence. Drug dependence may also occur in a more subtle manner and result in the seeking out of drugs for the pleasant and exciting sensations, and a feeling of well-being, that they may promote. This type of drug dependence, which is called *habituation,* is essentially recreational; a typical physical withdrawal illness does not occur in the absence of these drugs. It is also called *psychogenic (pyschic* or *psychologic) dependence*. Such drugs include the amphetamines, cocaine, hallucinogens, marihuana, nicotine (tobacco), caffeine, and, in small amounts, ethanol.

Drug abuse. The voluntary taking of drugs for nontherapeutic reasons is called drug abuse. The participants are sometimes referred to as compulsive drug users. The terms addict and addiction are old and popular ones that, it is said, are too imprecise for scientific use. The *Oxford English Dictionary* definition of an addict is "one who is addicted to the habitual and excessive use of a drug . . ." "Addicted" means "attached to ones own act." This definition appears to fit those who indulge in compulsive drug abuse. The dislike for the term addict may be due to its moral connotations rather than any scientific imprecision.

The therapeutic use of drugs may also result in drug dependence, and subsequently lead to drug abuse. Morphine and its analogues are used to relieve pain and ease the burdens of the dying. (The risks of addiction in the latter situation have been politically debated!) Barbiturates are used as sedatives, to promote sleep, and as anticonvulsants. Some patients even abhor the withdrawal of preparations of thyroid hormones and corticosteroids, and instances of their abuse have been reported. Nonnarcotic analgesic mixtures, especially those containing aspirin and phenacetin, have also been used for an alleged ability to promote a feeling of relaxation, and their abuse has resulted in virtual epidemics of kidney failure (analgesic nephropathy) in some communities.

Drug abuse can result in serious social, financial, and legal problems, not only for the participant but also for his or her friends and associates. It can also adversely affect health. Apart from the physical and mental anguish of the abstinence syndrome, drug abuse can result in illness, and even death, due to overdosage and the presence of toxic substances in the preparations that are used. Such accidents are not uncommon, especially as the composition and bioavailability of "street" drugs are not standardized according to pharmacopoeia-type criteria. The general social situation may even result in a predisposition to suicide. There are some relatively minor types of side effects, such as constipation and pinpoint pupils in morphine addicts; loss of appetite and necrosis of the nasal mucosa in those who snort cocaine; and the hangover in abusers of ethanol and barbiturates. Reproductive failure, including impotence, may occur, and nutritional disorders can result from a generally disordered life-style. Serious infections such as hepatitis can result from the use of nonsterile drug preparations and syringes.

Mechanisms of drug dependence and tolerance

Drug dependence is always associated with tolerance, though the converse does not necessarily occur. There is no universally accepted theory of the relatedness of drug tolerance to, and dependence on agents that depress the central nervous system. Several proposals have been made, however (see Clouet and Iwatsubo, 1975; Snyder, 1977; Collier, 1980). Some special properties of tolerance in association with physical drug dependence must be taken into account for any such hypotheses:

1. Physical dependence develops only in tissues that become tolerant to a drug; tolerance, however, is not always accompanied by dependence.
2. The tolerance and dependence are specific for a particular drug or the same chemical group of agonists. However, antagonist drugs of the same group may actually elicit withdrawal illness.
3. The phenomenon only occurs following a direct specific interaction of the tissue and the drug. If the drug is excluded from such sites by the presence of an antagonist, the development of tolerance and dependence can be prevented.
4. The processes may be initiated following a single exposure to a drug and may continue for a long time. Some relatively permanent change thus appears to become incorporated, or encoded, into the cell.
5. The physiological pattern of the effects of the abstinence syndrome are roughly opposite to those seen following the chronic administration of the drug itself. That is, there is general excitation, as opposed to depression, of the central nervous system.
6. The development of tolerance and physical dependence can be prevented experimentally by the presence of drugs that inhibit protein synthesis. Such drugs may act in several different ways such as a prevention of genetic transcription and translation. These observations are exciting as they offer a possible explanation as to how a "memory" of the drug exposure may be perpetuated and encoded into the cells. Changes in protein synthesis ("induction" theory) could be mediating changes in tissue enzyme levels, numbers of receptors, or even the formation of antibodies.
7. Tolerance and dependence have been associated with changes in the activity of the adenylate cyclase system. Morphine can block a stimulation of adenylate cyclase in vitro in brain tissue. In cultured brain cells morphine has been shown to initially inhibit adenylate cyclase; but subsequently, following chronic exposure, there is a compensatory increase in the levels of this enzyme.
8. A quasi morphine withdrawal syndrome can be elicited in rats by the administration of drugs that inhibit phosphodiesterase, an enzyme responsible for the inactivation of endogenous cyclic AMP.

It is generally considered that central depressant drugs, such as morphine and the barbiturates, bring about tolerance and dependence by influencing the functioning of neurotransmitters, which may excite or inhibit other nerve cells. They could be increasing or decreasing the release of such transmitters, be facilitating or blocking their actions, or be mimicking their effects. Such theories of drug dependence thus postulate that changes in the levels, effectiveness, or sensitivity to neurotransmitters, such as norepinephrine, 5-hydroxytryptamine, or endorphins, might be occurring.

One such neurohumoral adaptation theory of tolerance and physical dependence suggests that in response to a depressant drug there is an adaptational *rise in the levels of the neurotransmitter,* possibly occurring as a result of the increased synthesis of an enzyme involved in its biosynthesis. Such an effect would tend to overcome the depressant effects of the drug. However, when the drug is withdrawn, the elevated transmitter levels then result in a hyperexcitable state that is consistent with the abstinence syndrome. Despite numerous attempts, unequivocal evidence of such rises in neurotransmitter levels has not been forthcoming.

A second theory considers likely the involvement of a *negative feedback* control mechanism controlling some aspect of cellular responses to the drug and neurotransmitters. There are, however, several variations of this theme.

A recent variant involves the endorphins. These substances, which include the enkephalins, are peptides that have been identified in the brain and have morphine-like analgesic actions. Morphine appears to mimic their effects. Both types of compounds, the endogenous and exogenous ones, combine with the same opiate receptors, which have also been identified in the brain. When morphine is administered, it occupies opiate receptors that are unoccupied by the endorphins. In response, the adjacent endorphin-secreting neurons decrease their production of this neurotransmitter so that more morphine is needed to elicit an effect. Tolerance is thus observed. If the morphine is subsequently withdrawn, there is then insufficient endorphin for normal functioning of the tissue, and the withdrawal syndrome ensues. The decline in endorphin levels may be due to the induction of an enzyme that destroys it.

A third variation of the general principle of adaptational compensation of neurotransmitter functions involves the development of an increase in sensitivity, called *denervation supersensitivity.* There is in such a system no requirement for changes in neurotransmitter levels or their biosynthetic processes. The phenomenon of denervation supersensitivity is well known in peripheral tissues where it can be accomplished surgically or with drugs. According to this hypothesis, the presence of an inhibitory drug may result in an increased sensitivity at postsynaptic sites in nerve cells so that less neurotransmitter is needed to elicit a response. Higher doses of the inhibitory drug would be required, which can account for tolerance. When the drug is removed, however, the tissue will display a hyperexcitability in response to the usual, normal, level of the transmitter. The increase in sensitivity could involve an increase in the numbers of receptors at the postsynaptic site, but this possibility is not currently considered likely.

A fourth theory is concerned with changes in the activity of the *adenylate cyclase system,* which are clearly involved in the action of opioid drugs. One of the functions of cyclic AMP in the brain involves the control of the permeability of its cells to ions, such as Na. It is unknown, however, whether its presence in cells that are responsive to the central depressant drugs only reflects this function at such sites. Using cell cultures of brain neuroblastoma cells, it has been shown that morphine initially decreases the activity of adenylate cyclase, but with chronic exposure the amounts of the enzyme present in the cells increase (Sharma et al., 1975, 1977). When the morphine is removed, cyclic AMP production rises markedly, and this may account for the withdrawal syndrome. (This process is summarized in Figure 22.) It is possible that the changes in cyclic AMP levels are mediating a feedback inhibition mechanism that is controlling the production of the endorphins from the adjacent nerve cells. It is, however, uncertain at this time whether the phenomenon of dependence is occurring in the cell that contains the opiate receptors or is a function of adjoining cells, or both. The inhibition of the development of tolerance and dependence by inhibitors of protein synthesis could be blocking the induction of the enzymes involved in the compensatory mechanisms.

Drug interactions

When in the body, or even the medicine bottle, at the same time, two or more drugs may interact so that the response differs from that which each alone would exert. Such drug interactions may be either beneficial or harmful.

It is quite common for several drugs to be administered concurrently,

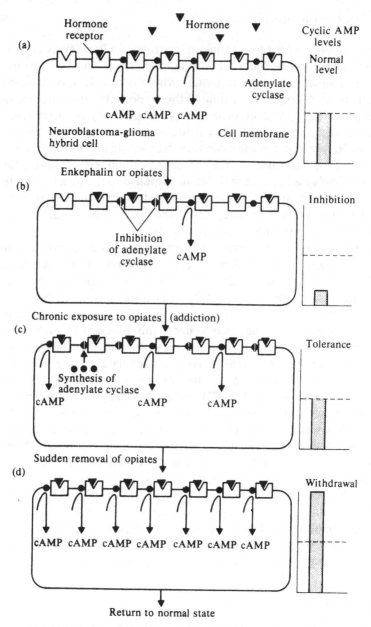

Figure 22. A diagrammatic summary of the effects of opioids, including morphine and the endorphins (enkephalins), on the adenylate cyclase system in a cultured cell line of nerve cells (neuroblastoma × glioma hybrid NG108-15). These observations provide a model for tolerance and addiction to opiates in man. (a) The adenylate cyclase can be stimulated by various substances, including hormones, so that there is an increase in the production of cyclic

and sometimes a whole host of them may be given together. There is considerable variation in this practice, some of which may reflect national and ethnic habits, and fashions. The results of an international survey showing the average number of drugs used on each patient after he or she had been admitted to the hospital, are shown in Table 6. The number used varied from about five in Scotland to nine in the United States. However, individual patients have been observed, in hospitals or elsewhere, who have been taking more than 30 different drugs at the same time. This general situation has been conservatively described as "multiple drug use," possibly less politely as "polypharmacy," and most realistically as "pharmacomania." The risk of an unfavorable drug interaction increases with the number of drugs used, so that such practices are generally to be abhorred. The reason for the profligacy may be a lack of awareness by the physician of the situation or the potential problems that may ensue. Multiple drug use can occur insidiously or accidentally owing to the simultaneous treatment of one patient by several physicians with different specialties, who may be unaware of each other's ministrations. In addition many drugs are freely

Table 6. *Extent of drug use during hospitalization in five countries*

Country	Number of patients monitored	Number of drugs given per admission
United States	9,097	9.1
Canada	1,182	7.2
Israel	1,706	6.6
New Zealand	619	5.8
Scotland	550	5.1

Source: Whiting and Goldberg (1977).

Caption to Fig. 22 (*cont.*)
AMP. (b) The acute administration of opioids, such as morphine or enkephalin (an endorphin), inhibits the adenyl cyclase so that the production of cyclic AMP declines. (c) On chronic exposure, however, there is a compensatory increase in the synthesis of adenyl cyclase or a conversion from a low to high activity form, so that cyclic AMP production returns toward normal levels. This process can be blocked by cycloheximide, which inhibits protein synthesis. This is the stage where tolerance occurs. (d) If the opioids are suddenly withdrawn, the uninhibited adenyl cyclase produces excessive amounts of cyclic AMP. This response may trigger the withdrawal syndrome. (From Snyder, 1977; based on the results of Sharma, Klee and Nirenberg, 1975. Copyright 1977 by *Scientific American*, Inc. All rights reserved)

available without prescription, and some people have a penchant to indulge in their use.

Mechanisms of drug interactions

Drugs may interact with each other in various ways, both in the body (in vivo) and outside of it (in vitro), in medicine bottles, syringes, and intravenous infusion solutions. *Pharmaceutical incompatibility* (in vitro) refers to the interactions of drugs that occur during storage or in administering devices, and usually involves chemical reactions that may result in the precipitation or inactivation of one or both drugs. Drugs that are to be mixed prior to administration thus should be checked to see that they are mutually compatible in the solution being used. Tetracycline antibiotics (as their hydrochlorides) and hydrocortisone sodium succinate thus mutually precipitate each other in solution. Mixing some types of penicillin preparations with gentamicin results in the inactivation of the latter.

Interactions in the body (in vivo) refers to the influence of one drug on the action of another such drug by either pharmacokinetic or pharmacodynamic means. In a *pharmacokinetic* type of interaction, accessibility to the ultimate site of action may be altered. This alteration may result from changes in the absorption of the drug from the gut, its binding to plasma proteins, or its elimination as a result of the functioning of the liver and kidneys. A *pharmacodynamic type* of interaction is said to occur when the drug's action directly involves the response of the effector system or end organ.

Pharmacokinetic interactions. The roles of absorption, plasma protein binding, biotransformation, and excretion in the actions of drugs were described in Chapter 6. Any of these processes may have a role in drug interactions.

One drug may alter the *absorption,* from the gut or an injection site, of another drug. The antacid aluminum hydroxide binds tetracycline antibiotics and so may prevent their attaining effective therapeutic levels in the blood. Cholestyramine binds bile acids in the gut and is used to reduce plasma lipid levels, but it can also bind drugs such as thyroxine and anticoagulants, and so reduces their effectiveness. This action of cholestyramine can also be used to enhance the elimination of cardiac glycosides in patients suffering from digitalis toxicity.

Many drugs can be *bound to plasma proteins* where they may share common or adjacent binding sites. Thus, one drug may displace or exclude another from binding so that the "free," pharmacologically active, levels change (see Chapter 6, under "Distribution and binding of drugs"). For instance, the antiinflammatory drug phenylbutazone and oral anticoagulants, such as warfarin, mutually compete, so that the free levels of warfarin may rise, and hemorrhage can result.

The *biotransformation* of drugs to other compounds, which may be more or less active than the parent one, occurs principally in the liver (see Chapter 6, under "Metabolism, or biotransformation, of drugs"). The hepatic microsomal enzymes can be increased or induced, as a result of the actions of many drugs and chemicals, including barbiturates, phenytoin, ethanol, and cigarette smoke. On the other hand, the activities of hepatic enzymes can also be inhibited by many drugs, such as phenelzine, which inhibits monoamine oxidase in the liver, and elsewhere. The responses to drugs that are inactivated, or activated by such enzymes may, obviously, be influenced by the presence of drugs that thus affect their metabolism.

Excretion of drugs and their metabolites in the urine depends on their filtration across the glomerulus, secretion across the wall of the renal tubule, and reabsorption from the filtrate. Drugs frequently compete for transport by the tubular secretory mechanism and so may interfere with each other's elimination. The most famous example is the use of probenicid to block excretion of penicillin, thus increasing the latter's effectiveness (see later in this section). Because many drugs are weak acids or weak bases, the pH of the urine will influence their ionization and hence their reabsorption. Examples are salicylates and barbiturates, which are weak acids, and amphetamine, which is a weak base. Some drugs such as the diuretics and antacids may alter the pH of the urine so that interactions involving excretion with the above types of drugs may occur.

Pharmacodynamic interactions. Interactions that occur as a result of the responses of the effector system to the drugs involve several types of processes.

Two drugs may both interact with an identical receptor in the effector organ. They may thus mutually enhance the response or reduce it, depending on whether two agonists or an agonist and an antagonist are present.

Opioid drugs, such as morphine and heroin, can, in excess, result in death from respiratory depression. This adverse response is mediated by the action of these narcotics on the respiratory center in the brain stem. Competitive antagonists can, however, block their effects. Naloxone is such a drug, which is used therapeutically to help maintain respiration in morphine and heroin poisoning. It can also result in withdrawal effects (see preceding section, "Tachyphylaxis, tolerance, and dependence"). Other opioid agonists such as codeine and pethidine may, on the other hand, increase the respiratory depression.

Two drugs may influence a response by acting at different types of receptor sites, which may be capable of engendering either similar or opposing effects. Such parallel receptor sites may both be present in the same organ, though they act by different mechanisms. Thus, the relaxation of smooth muscle in blood vessels may be enhanced by drugs that either block its α-adrenergic receptors (which normally mediate contraction) or by a direct action on the muscle cells themselves. The latter effects are seen with some hypotensive drugs (e.g., hydralazine and diazoxide). Thus the two types of drugs acting together may produce a greater overall response than either alone can elicit.

In other instances the different types of receptor sites may be even farther apart and be present in separate tissues. Drugs with such relatively distant, but still parallel, types of actions can also antagonize or reinforce each other's effects. To use the example of regulation of blood pressure once more: Dilatation in one vascular bed, such as skeletal muscle (β-adrenergic receptors), may oppose a rise in blood pressure due to a constriction in more peripheral blood vessels (α-adrenergic receptors). Different types of drugs that depress brain functions may also reinforce each other's effect, though they utilize different mechanisms. Thus it can be dangerous to engage in ethanol drinking while taking other drugs such as morphine, barbiturates, and antihistamines. All of these drugs can interact with each other to produce an overall toxic response. However, their primary sites of action in the brain differ.

The physiological environment of the effector organs may be altered by a drug so that the response to another one is increased or decreased. Antiinflammatory drugs, such as phenylbutazone and indomethacin, produce as a side effect sodium and fluid retention. This effect can reduce the response to antihypertensive drugs. Diuretic drugs can influence the excretion of potassium in the urine. Thiazides, furosemide, and ethacrynic acid all increase urinary potassium loss and so can produce a hypokalemia. These lowered plasma K levels increase the effects of cardiac glycoside drugs, such as digoxin, so that a dose that is therapeutically correct at normal plasma K levels may then exert toxic actions. Such a loss of K can also result in cardiac arrhythmias and so antagonize the desired effects of antiarrhythmic drugs, such as lidocaine and procainamide.

Beneficial effects of drug interactions

It is often thought that drug interactions are mostly harmful but this is not so, as two or more drugs are often used to advantage to treat a disease. There can be several aims and strategies in the combined use of such drugs.

Drug combinations can block, or compensate for, undesirable side effects, toxicity, or poisoning. Many antihypertensive drugs, apart from lowering the blood pressure, also produce a retention of sodium resulting in the accumulation of edema fluid in the body. This side effect, apart from possibly being cosmetically distressing, reduces the effectiveness of the drug in lowering blood pressure. Thus, in many patients with hypertension diuretic drugs are also administered to promote urinary Na loss. Such drugs, which include the thiazides and furosemide, also have an ability of their own to lower blood pressure, which may be additive to that of the original hypotensive drug.

Hydralazine is an antihypertensive drug that acts by dilating peripheral blood vessels. As a result, a reflex increase in heart rate occurs (tachycardia). In order to overcome this side effect, the β-adrenergic antagonist propranolol can be given to help block this reflex. Propranolol also has a hypotensive effect of its own which is also additive to that of the hydralazine. A diuretic may be added to this regimen to compensate for the fluid retention, which is also associated with the use of the hydralazine.

Drugs may be used in attempts to overcome acute toxicity and poisoning by other drugs. Acute toxicity due to the salicylate drug aspirin is quite common, especially in children. Salicylates are weak acids so that their excretion in the urine is increased when the urine is alkaline, as the drug is ionized and cannot be reabsorbed across the renal tubule wall. The administration of sodium bicarbonate makes the urine alkaline and can be used to hasten the elimination of the drug. Conversely, ammonium chloride, which acidifies the urine, can be used to promote the excretion of amphetamines, which are weak bases.

Two drugs, each of which can elicit the same type of effect, can be used in the same individual to increase a therapeutic effect. Such a combination may result in an additive effect of two drugs by an action on the same or parallel effectors. It may also result in the potentiation of the overall effect.

The combined effect of two types of antihypertensive drugs (discussed above in this section) is commonly employed in the treatment of hypertension. Another rationale for using two different antihypertensive drugs at the same time is that the blood pressure may be controlled while using a dose of each drug that is low enough to reduce the possibility of side effects from each.

One drug may potentiate or increase the effectiveness of another drug while having no such endogenous action of its own. Some local anesthetics, such as procaine, are often prepared in solutions that contain epinephrine. The latter substance constricts peripheral blood vessels so that when the procaine is injected into tissues, it is less rapidly dispersed from the site than usual. Its action is thus prolonged. Procaine can also be toxic, so that there is the additional advantage that blood levels of the drug will rise less rapidly. When penicillin first became available in World War II, its supplies were limited. Following its administration, its levels in the blood decline, largely as a result of its active secretion across the wall of the renal tubule into the urine. In order to reduce this excretion of the penicillin, and so facilitate its action in the body, it was administered together with probenicid, which is excreted in the same manner. By competing with the penicillin for a place on the renal tubular secreting pump mechanism, the probenicid delays the fall in blood penicillin levels and so enhances its effects.

Harmful effects of drug interactions

It has been estimated that of the total number of adverse effects of drugs, 7 to 22 percent are due to their interaction with other drugs. Some examples of the nature of such effects, the drugs that cause them and their mechanisms are summarized in Table 7.

Table 7. *Some examples of adverse effects of drug interactions*

Response	Drugs	Mechanism
Bleeding and hemorrhage	Dicumarol and tolbutamide	Mutual displacement from binding to plasma proteins
	Dicumarol and phenylbutazone	Displacement from binding and decreased hepatic metabolism
Hypertension	MAO antidepressants (e.g., phenelzine) and amines (e.g., amphetamine and phenylephrine)	Blockade of amine destruction
	Guanethidine and tricyclic antidepressants (e.g., imipramine and amitryptyline)	Loss of control of hypertension due to blockade of uptake of guanethidine into nerve terminals
	Guanethidine and phenylbutazone	Reduction of guanethidine effect by Na retention
Heartbeat irregular	Digitalis and thiazide diuretics	Lowering of plasma K by diuretics; heart sensitized
	Procainamide and lidocaine, and thiazide diuretics	Lowering of plasma K by diuretics; heart sensitized
Respiratory depression (central)	Narcotic analgesics, ethanol, barbiturates, chlorpromazine	Mutual toxicities
Respiratory paralysis (peripheral)	Succinylcholine and cholinesterase inhibitors (e.g., ecothiophate, DFP)	Blockade of inactivation by cholinesterase
	Tubocurarine and aminoglycoside antibiotics	Potentiation of effect
Deafness	Ethacrynic acid and aminoglycoside antibiotics	Mutual toxicity
Hypoglycemia	Insulin and propranolol	Blockade of compensatory responses
	Tolbutamide and phenylbutazone	Displacement from binding and inhibition of drugs' metabolism
	Tolbutamide and ethanol	Mutual hypoglycemic effects
Hyperglycemia	Tolbutamide, and diazoxide and thiazide diuretics	Antagonism of insulin release by diazoxide and thiazides
Lacticacidosis	Phenformin and ethanol	Mutual toxicity
Renal papillary necrosis (analgesic nephropathy)	Phenacetin and other nonnarcotic analgesics	?
Uric acid retention	Uricosuric drugs and salicylates (small doses)	Opposite actions

Adverse reactions to drugs

Chemicals can only be used as drugs when they have a preferential or selective action on certain tissues and organs in which it is hoped that some therapeutic response will be elicited. This selectivity, however, is only relative; most drugs become widely dispersed in the body and thus can gain access to many sites where they may also have undesirable effects. Such adverse responses to drugs are described as side effects and as toxic reactions.

Side effects are usually taken to mean relatively minor, non-life-threatening, effects, which are usually acceptable in relation to the seriousness of the disease being treated. For instance, some discomfort may be experienced, such as indigestion, nausea and even vomiting, diarrhea, constipation, sleepiness, and confusion. Such effects may decline with the continued use of the drug, or they may be tolerated. Sometimes side effects of drugs can be reduced by decreasing the dose, dividing it into smaller parts, or administering it at certain times, such as before or after meals. Other side effects can, however, be more distressing and inconvenient, such as the postural hypotension that is commonly associated with the use of many antihypertensive drugs, and the fluid retention that may result from taking oral contraceptive drugs.

Toxic reactions to drugs are more serious and may be debilitating or even fatal. In everyday parlance, they are synonomous with poisoning. In some instances, however, a serious toxic type of reaction may even be acceptable therapeutically. For instance, the antifungal agent amphotericin B is one of the few drugs that can be effective in the treatment of systemic fungal infections. Such diseases have a high risk of mortality; so although the drug can have very serious adverse effects on the kidney (see Chapter 10) and other tissues, which can be fatal, it is still used, though carefully and only in hospital patients.

The separation of the adverse effects of drugs into categories of side effects and toxicities is thus somewhat arbitrary.

Occurrence

Serious adverse reactions to drugs account for about 5 percent of all hospital admissions in the United States. It has also been estimated that about 10 percent of hospitalized patients experience such undesired drug effects. To these individuals must be added the hosts of other users of drugs who have more minor, but largely unavoidable, adverse symptoms from the drugs they take. Adverse reactions, if they occur, often are apparent soon after a patient starts taking a drug; however, in some instances such a response may arise only in certain circumstances, such as the subsequent onset of another disease or following long-term exposure. An adverse response may even be delayed for many years, after the use of the drug has ceased; carcinogenic effects are the best known examples, and the most feared.

Causes and predisposing factors

Size of dose. Adverse reactions to drugs are related to the size of the dose. Thus, drugs that have a high therapeutic index, or margin of safety, are less likely to have toxic effects at therapeutically effective doses. In other instances, however, the balance may be more delicate. It should also be remembered that overdosage can occur chronically, over a long period of time, if the drug can accumulate in the body. Overdose can also occur by medical error, accident, or attempts at self-destruction. As described elsewhere (Chapter 4) all preparations of the same drug are not absorbed uniformly. Therefore in changing from one type or brand to another, an unpredictable difference in absorption may be observed, and produce adverse effects.

Chemical nature of the drug. The chemical nature of the drug itself is obviously a major factor in determining its side effects and toxicity. Many types of drugs have well-recognized, rather general effects on physiological mechanisms, which may be widely dispersed in the body. Thus, a desired therapeutic action on one organ may be difficult to isolate from an accompanying effect on another organ. A drug such as propranolol, which has a general β-adrenergic blocking effect, will, not surprisingly, have a number of different effects associated with different organ systems. Propranolol is widely used to treat hypertension; however, β-adrenergic mechanisms also help control the contractility of the heart, the relaxation of the bronchi, and the mobilization of glucose from glycogen. The use of this drug to treat hypertension may thus be inappropriate in patients who also suffer from heart disease, asthma, or diabetes mellitus.

A chemical group in a molecule may be associated with a certain type of toxicity, and if this association is recognized, it may be possible to remove such a moiety or substitute for it. Carbutamide was a prototype oral hypoglycemic antidiabetic drug whose early use was associated with an unacceptably frequent occurrence of agranulocytosis. This usually fatal toxicity, involving the white blood cells, was related to the presence of an amino group in the drug molecule. When a methyl group was substituted for the amino group, to produce tolbutamide, this adverse effect was virtually eliminated.

The blood–brain barrier limits the movement of many drugs from the plasma to the central nervous system; drugs that can pass across this barrier are quite likely to exert adverse effects that are of a neurological nature. This facility to cross the blood–brain barrier is a function of chemical structure. Thus the antihypertensive drug α-methyldopa can enter the brain, where it may exert its hypotensive action, but at this site it also has marked sedative effects, which can limit its dosage. Guanethidine, on the other hand, cannot gain access to the brain and so has a strong hypotensive action, which is, notably, without direct neurological types of side effects.

Condition of the patient. The condition of the patient may have a determining role in the initiation of adverse reactions to a drug.

Age may be important. The very young and the elderly are usually more sensitive to drugs than other patients. The differences they exhibit in comparison to more mature children and younger adults mainly reflect underdeveloped or declining physiological systems.

The *sex* may be important; men and women can respond differently to drugs. In women adverse reactions are reported more frequently, and are also a more common cause of death than in men. Pregnancy is a woman's condition, and the resulting physiological changes may influence drug therapy. Adjustments of dosage and changes in the drugs used may be necessary. Possible risks to the fetus must be considered, and in view of the possibility of teratogenic effects of drugs in early pregnancy (see later in this section, under "Teratogenic effects of drugs") they are then used with caution, if at all.

Diet may influence the response to a drug. Thus, malnutrition may result in a decline in plasma protein levels and hence reduce the potential sites for the binding of drugs. Substances may also be obtained in the food that interact with drugs; for instance, tyramine in the presence of antidepressant drugs that inhibit monoamine oxidase can result in hypertension and even cerebral hemorrhage. The contents of the gastrointestinal tract can also influence the absorption of drugs into the blood.

The *concurrent use of other drugs and chemicals* for therapy or pleasure may promote adverse effects. The problems that may arise from the use of oral contraceptives in women who smoke are described later in this chapter, under "Drugs and environmental chemicals." Ethanol drinking can also modify the actions of many drugs, and, apart from those effects that also act on the brain, it can precipitate lactic acidosis in those using the antidiabetic drug phenformin, and a hypoglycemia in users of insulin. Adverse reactions due to interactions with other drugs are an important determinant of adverse responses (see under "Drug interactions," preceding section).

Unpredictable, *idiosyncratic* responses and adverse reactions may occur, which reflect the particular genetic constitution of the individual (see "Genetic differences in drug responses," earlier in this chapter). *Allergies* to some drugs may also develop in certain people (see below, subsection on "Drug allergy").

The presence of concurrent *diseases* can have important effects on a person's responses to drugs. Biotransformation and excretion of drugs largely depend on adequate functioning of the liver and kidneys (see Chapter 6, under "Metabolism, or biotransformation, of drugs" and "Excretion of drugs"). Thus, toxicities to drugs are more likely to occur in liver and kidney diseases because of the accumulation in the body of a drug or its metabolites. In addition some diseases may make certain tissues and organs more *sensitive* to the actions of drugs. As described earlier in this section, β-adrenergic blockade with pro-pranolol may worsen cardiac function in patients with congestive heart failure or result in bronchospasm in asthmatics. Aspirin may result in hemorrhage in patients with peptic ulcer or bleeding disorders. Oral contraceptives may increase the blood pressure to unacceptable levels in women with a minor degree of hypertension.

Nature of adverse reactions to drugs

The toxic and side effects of drugs may be manifested on any tissue, organ, or metabolic system in the body. Some examples of the nature of such disorders are summarized in Table 8. Procedures for monitoring adverse drug reactions are described later in this section, under "Monitoring and evaluation of adverse effects of drugs."

Drug allergy

Allergic responses to drugs are uncommon, but when they occur they are usually serious, and may even be fatal. These adverse responses to drugs can occur following the administration of very small

Table 8. *Nature of some adverse reactions to drugs*

Site of action	Nature of response	Example of drug
Gastrointestinal tract	Nausea, loss of appetite, vomiting	Many drugs, including cardiac glycosides
	Diarrhea	α-Adrenergic blockers, many antibiotics
	Constipation	Morphine, Fe, belladona alkaloids
	Peptic ulcer	Antiinflammatory drugs, reserpine
	Colitis	Clindamycin
	Malabsorption	Fe, mineral oil, tetracycline
Blood	Aplastic anemia	Chloramphenicol, indomethacin
	Agranulocytosis	Phenylbutazone, cytotoxic drugs
	Hemolytic anemia	Penicillin, α-methyldopa
	Thrombocytopenia	Cytotoxic drugs, phenylbutazone
	Thrombophlebitis	Oral contraceptives, estrogens
	Bleeding	Aspirin, anticoagulents
Liver	Necrosis	Acetaminophen (poisoning), methotrexate
	Cholestasis, jaundice	Oral contraceptives, chlorpropamide
	Tumors	Androgens, α-methyldopa, chlorpromazine
Kidney	Papillary necrosis	Nonnarcotic analgesics (phenacetin)
	Nephrotoxic (tubule)	Amphotericin B, *cis*-Pt, Hg
	Renal stones	Acetazolamide
	Resistance to ADH	Lithium, demeclocycline
Respiratory system	Depressed breathing	Central action: opioid drugs, ethanol, barbiturates
		Peripheral action: tubocurarine, succinylcholine, streptomycin
	Bronchospasm	Drugs causing allergic reactions, β-adrenergic blockers (propranolol)
Cardiovascular system		
Heartbeat	Tachycardia	Hydralazine, diazoxide, amphetamine, atropine
	Bradycardia	Cholinergic drugs, propranolol
	Ventricular fibrillation	Cardiac glycosides
	Heart block	Quinidine, procainamide, propranolol
Heart contraction	Depression	Quinidine, procainamide

Table 8. (*cont.*)

Site of action	Nature of response	Example of drug
Blood pressure	Hypotension	Drugs causing allergic reactions, prazosin (initial response), anti-anginal drugs, chlorpromazine
Central nervous system	Sleepiness, sedation	α-Methyldopa, antihistamines
	Dreams, nightmares	Propranolol, α-methyldopa
	Confusion, hallucinations, delirium	Cimetidine, digitalis, pentazocine, isoniazid
	Depression	Reserpine, corticosteroids, L-dopa, indomethacin
	Euphoria	Corticosteroids, L-dopa
	Tremor	L-Dopa, antipsychotic drugs
	Encephalopathy	Al(OH)$_3$ (in renal failure)
	Extrapyramidal reactions	Reserpine, L-dopa, α-methyldopa, chlorpromazine
Eye	Glaucoma	Corticosteroids, atropine
	Cataracts	Corticosteroids, ecothiophate
Ear	Deafness and tinnitus	Ethacrynic acid, aminoglycoside antibiotics, salicylates, quinidine
Reproductive system: male	Impotence	α-Adrenergic blocking hypotensive drugs, estrogens, narcotics
	Gynecomastia	Cardiac glycosides, cimetidine, spironolactone, estrogens
Reproductive system: female	Galactorrhea	Phenothiazines, reserpine, α-methyldopa, estrogens
	Amenorrhea	Oral contraceptives, reserpine, morphine, chlorpromazine
	Virilization	Androgenic steroids
	Menorrhagia	Anticoagulants
Endocrine glands	B-cells, islets of Langerhans	Inhibition: thiazide diuretics, diazoxide
	Adenohypophysis	Prolactinemia: reserpine, α-methyldopa; inhibition of ACTH release: corticosteroids
	Neurohypophysis	Inhibition of ADH release: ethanol, chloral hydrate Increase of ADH release: ether, carbamazepine, vincristine, morphine, smoking

Table 8. (*cont.*)

Site of action	Nature of response	Example of drug
	Thyroid	Inhibition: lithium, Na-nitroprusside
Skin	Allergic responses, eczema, etc.	Many drugs
	Alopecia	Vitamin A, cytotoxic drugs
	Acne	Androgens, corticosteroids
	Discoloration and pigmentation	Quinacrine, corticotropin, chlorpromazine
	Thinning and rosacea	Topical corticosteroids
Immune system	Increased risk of infection	Cytotoxic drugs, corti-costeroids
Intermediary metabolism	Hyperglycemia or decline in glucose tolerance	Corticosteroids, diazoxide, oral contraceptives, thiazides
	Hypoglycemia	Propranolol (with insulin), ethanol, insulin and oral antidiabetic overdose
	Lactic acidosis	Phenformin, ethanol
	Hyperuricemia	Salicylates (small dose), thiazides
	Growth inhibition	Corticosteroids, andro-gens, estrogens
Mineral metabolism	Sodium retention	Corticosteroids, phenyl-butazone, carbenoxo-lone, antihypertensives, antacids
	Sodium loss	Amphotericin B
	Potassium retention	Spironolactone, K-supple-ments, amiloride
	Potassium loss	Thiazide diuretics, furosemide, ampho-tericin B, corticoster-oids, laxatives
Hydrogen, bicarbonate metabolism	Metabolic alkalosis	Many diuretics, $NaHCO_3$ (as antacid)
	Metabolic acidosis	Acetazolamide, salicylate intoxication
Calcium metabolism	Osteoporosis	Corticosteroids
	Osteomalacia	Anticonvulsants (e.g., phenytoin)
	Hypercalcemia	Vitamin D overdose, thiazides
Phosphate metabolism	Loss of phosphate	$Al(OH)_3$ (antacid)

doses; for instance, a single penicillin tablet. Hence they can occur inadvertently, as when ill-labelled proprietary mixtures of drugs are administered. Such responses are often the result of an antigen–antibody interaction, which can lead to the release of toxic constituents from cells, such as histamine, or may damage or kill the cells. The ability of a drug to act as an antigen and promote the formation of an antibody depends on several factors. Most drugs alone are not antigenic, with the exceptions of foreign proteins and large peptides such as hormone preparations made from the endocrine glands of animals. To be antigenic most drugs must bind covalently to macromolecules such as proteins, in the body. Such a drug itself, however, is not necessarily the antigenic component of a medicine; one of its metabolites may be the active agent, or the activity may be due to impurities that are present. The latter may reflect inadequacies in the manufacturing or purification procedures. For instance, the antigenic effects of penicillin were once the result of the presence of foreign proteins that remained with the drug following its preparation by a microbial fermentation process. Remnants of cattle or pig proinsulins (the C-peptide) are major contributors to the antigenic properties of many insulin preparations. The method of administration may also influence the occurrence of allergies; they are, for instance, more common following topical and parenteral use than when given orally. There also appears to be a predisposing genetic component because certain individuals and their relatives are more prone to develop drug allergies than other persons.

Prediction of the likely occurrence of allergies can be difficult. Although theoretically it must follow at least a single exposure to the drug, such an event cannot always be readily identified, even though an allergic response has been observed. It may also occur rather unexpectedly, after several courses of treatment. Sensitization may depend on the size of the dose used. Drug allergies are less common in children than adults. Allergy is usually quite specific to a single drug; however, cross-reactions involving two different, but usually chemically related, drugs may occur. From empirical observations certain drugs are known to have the potential ability to cause certain types of allergic responses.

In order to produce an allergic response the drug-related antigen must be able to react in some way so as to disturb the functioning of cells. Allergic reactions have been categorized as anaphylactic reactions, blood cell destruction, serum sickness, and skin reactions (Coombs-Gell types I to IV).

Anaphylactic reactions (type I) may occur within minutes of the administration of a drug, such as penicillin, and are often fatal. They result from the release of histamine from sensitized mast cells, which have the antibody on their surface. The histamine can produce a bronchospasm and drop in blood pressure leading to asphyxiation, shock, and widespread edema.

Destruction of blood cells and platelets may occur when the antigen attaches itself to the surface of the cells, and these cells are killed following an interaction with circulating antibodies (type II, cytotoxic). Such blood dyscrasias include:

1. Hemolytic anemia, as in response to the antiarrhythmic drug quinidine, and the hypotensive agent α-methyldopa (an autoimmune type of response).
2. Agranulocytosis, which can occur with the antiinflammatory drug phenylbutazone and propylthiouracil, an antithyroid drug.
3. Thrombocytopenia, which may result from use of the antimalarial drug quinine and thiazide diuretics.

Serum sickness may occur because of the binding of circulating antigen–antibody complexes to the wall of blood vessels, resulting in their inflammation (type III). A number of antimicrobial drugs, including the sulfonamides, penicillin and streptomycin, and the thiouracils, may initiate this type of adverse reaction.

Skin reactions and rashes of the delayed hypersensitivity type (IV) may occur owing to the release of antibodies from sensitized T-lymphocytes. Such reactions may occur in response to penicillin, topical neomycin, and local anesthetics. Skin reactions may, however, also occur in response to other mechanisms (types) of drug allergy.

Carcinogenic Actions of Drugs

It is widely considered that 70 to 90 percent of the malignant tumors that occur in man are the result of exposure to environmental agents, including chemicals (see Weisburger, 1978; Fraumeni, 1979; Ames, 1979). In man about 40 percent of cancer may be due to smoking. There is concern that drugs used therapeutically may contribute to such environmentally caused cancers, especially because many appear to be quite exotic chemicals, some are cytotoxic, they may be concentrated in certain organs, such as the liver, kidneys, and urinary bladder, and exposure may occur for prolonged periods of time. For instance, antihypertensive drugs, oral antidiabetic agents, oral contraceptives, and antidepressive drugs and tranquilizers may be taken chronically for several decades of a person's lifetime. It is therefore a requirement that new drugs be tested for possible carcinogenic effects, using animals and microorganisms as models. Usually two species, such as rats and mice, are used in such animal tests, and they are given regular, usually sub-toxic, doses, if possible by a comparable route to that used in man, over their lifetimes. The animals are routinely examined for the occur-rence of tumors (see Goldberg, 1973). Some "old" drugs, which were introduced before such tests became obligatory, have been examined in this way, including the antidiabetic drugs tolbutamide and phenformin. (In these instances the animal tests were negative.) Many carcinogenic chemicals and drugs have been shown to have mutagenic effects on microorganisms, and such responses can be conveniently used to screen such substances for possible carcinogenic actions. Such a test using mutant strains of *Salmonella typhimurium,* the Ames test, is now widely used for screening drugs. Many epidemiological surveys have also been carried out in man on such drugs as oral contraceptives and antihypertensive agents. No evidence for carcinogenic effects of the former were noted, but at least one antihypertensive drug, reserpine, has been somewhat suspect.

Surprisingly few drugs have been shown to have carcinogenic effects in man. It has been estimated that drugs may account for 2 to 3 percent of environmentally produced cancers. Many drugs that have been shown to be carcinogenic in animals apparently do not have such ef-fects in man. Some drugs whose carcinogenic actions in man are usu-ally considered to be conclusive are: diethylstilbestrol (DES), which has female sex hormone (estrogenic) actions, and some cytotoxic and immunosuppressive drugs, including cyclophosphamide, which are used to treat some types of cancer and are used in kidney transplant procedures. On the basis of limited epidemiological surveys and/or animal studies, certain other drugs are considered suspect by some investigators. Apart from reserpine (which may be associated with breast cancer in women), this group includes phenacetin (a now un-popular analgesic, which may cause cancer of the renal papilla), an-drogenic anabolic steroids (which cause liver cancer), chloramphenicol (an antibiotic), and phenytoin (an anticonvulsant).

Mechanisms of carcinogenesis. Drugs and chemicals may exert carcinogenic effects via several types of mechanisms. The direct car-cinogenic effect itself is considered to be the result of the action of a substance called an *initiator,* which binds covalently to some cell component such as DNA, RNA, or a protein. This event may result in the death of the cell, but sometimes a mutation (genotoxic), resulting in an inherited error in the replication process of the cell, occurs. A mutant clone of cells is thus produced which may divide in an uncontrolled manner.

A drug or chemical that precipitates the formation of a malignant tumor may act in several ways:

1. It may exert a *direct effect* and combine with the susceptible cell component while in the same chemical form in which it was originally administered.
2. Alternatively, it may first require chemical modification, which occurs as a result of its metabolism in the body. It is then said to have an *indirect action*.
3. An interaction may occur between drugs and chemicals so that they both may contribute to the response. They are then said to have *cocarcinogenic effects*. Thus 75 percent of mouth cancers are known to occur in smokers who also drink alcohol.

Causes of cocarcinogenic effects. There are several possible reasons for interactions that produce cocarcinogenic effects. First, one drug or chemical may *facilitate the absorption* of another. Second, the *induction of liver enzymes,* such as may occur in response to smoking, pesticides and barbiturates, may enhance the conversion of an inactive form of a carcinogen to its active form.

It should, however, be noted that such a process may also result in an increased rate of inactivation of potential carcinogens, so that some drugs and chemicals could be exerting a protective action in the body. It is considered that such effects may normally be very important in protecting people against the carcinogenic effects of chemicals obtained from the external environment. Natural substances, such as we may acquire in our diet, could be acting to alter the metabolism of potential carcinogens. Such an interaction is considered to be an example of xenobiosis, and the participating nutrients are called *xenobiotics*. The artificial promotion of such a process of inactivation of carcinogens is a possible strategy for cancer prophylaxis.

Third, some substances may *increase the effectiveness of a carcinogen* subsequent to its action on the cell. Such cocarcinogenic chemicals are called *promoters*. They act by stimulating the proliferation of tissues so that the replication of the mutant cells is enhanced. Hormones and hormone-like drugs may act in this manner. Thus estrogens, such as diethylstilbestrol, increase the proliferation of uterine endometrial cells, an action that may account for the association of DES with the cancer of this tissue that occurs in women. On the other hand, it is also possible that the availability of a large number of appropriately dividing cells may offer a more susceptible environment for a cancer initiator to act.

Drugs that kill cells (cytotoxic) may indirectly, by *fostering the process of their replacement,* increase the chances of an error in DNA replication being perpetuated.

A process of *repair of damaged DNA* may be impaired by another drug.

Teratogenic effects of drugs

Congenital morphological abnormalities in man and animals have been a recorded source of curiosity for more than 2000 years (see Clegg, 1971; Wilson, 1974; Tuchmann-Duplessis, 1975). In man they are currently estimated to occur in about 5 percent of live births. About half of these defects are major, or gross, morphological deformities, whereas the others are less apparent, and some may be manifested as physiological or even behavioral abnormalities or differences. About half such disorders only become apparent several months after birth. The science of teratology (from a Greek word meaning monster) was defined and named in 1837 by I. Geoffrey Saint Hilaire, and then referred to major deformities such as phocomelia, anencephalia, and cleft palate. Drugs and chemicals that may cause such deformities are usually called teratogens. It has, however, been suggested (Tuchmann-Duplessis, 1975) that *dysmorphogens* would be a more appropriate term to use, to include all such substances that cause disorders, both major and minor.

The recent revival of interest in the subject of congenital deformities is partly the result of an observed iatrogenic teratogenesis. As described later in this chapter, under "The development of new drugs," the sedative-hypnotic drug thalidomide was observed in 1961 to produce phocomelia in the infants of mothers who took it in early pregnancy. Drugs and chemicals are, however, only one of several possible causes of congenital deformities, which may also result from genetic and chromosomal abnormalities, X-radiation, maternal infections, such as rubella, and nutritional disorders that may involve minerals, vitamins, and amino acids. Environmental contaminants from industrial wastes, such as methyl mercury, may also be teratogenic.

In animal experiments several hundred chemicals have been shown to exert teratogenic effects, including representatives of virtually all the main groups of drugs: cytotoxic agents, antibiotics, anesthetics, hypoglycemics, antihistamines, tranquilizers, corticosteroids, and salicylates. In animal tests such drugs are usually administered at relatively high doses compared to those used therapeutically in man. Thus it is probably not surprising to observe that they have not all been shown to have such an action in man, where, indeed, the number of unequivocal teratogenic drugs is quite small. Apart from thalidomide, it includes androgenic and estrogenic hormone-like preparations and folic acid antagonists. Epidemiological studies, in conjunction with animal tests, have on occasion suggested that other drugs may be teratogenic in man, including the anticonvulsant phenytoin, alkylating agents, like cyclophosphamide, ethanol, antihistaminic drugs, and even aspirin; but none of these suspicions has been confirmed.

Factors influencing teratogenic action. Several factors may influence the ability of a drug to exert a teratogenic action:

1. The *size of the dose* is important; as seen from animal tests, large numbers of drugs may be teratogenic, provided they are given in large enough doses.

2. The effect on the embryo is usually precisely related to *the drug's structure* rather than the general structure of the chemical family to which it belongs. No relationship appears to exist between the drug's pharmacodynamic and toxic actions and its teratogenic effect. For instance, analogues of thalidomide are not all teratogenic. Structure, of course, is important in relationship to the ability of the drug to cross the placenta.

3. The *developmental stage* when the embryo or fetus is exposed to the drug will determine its particular teratogenic effects. Pregnant women are especially sensitive from the 17th to the 42nd day after conception, at the end of which time organogenesis has nearly been completed. However, the developing external genitalia are susceptible for about 4 months, whereas the endocrine and nervous system are sensitive throughout pregnancy. The particular abnormality that occurs in response to a drug is related to the specific time in the pregnancy when exposure to its occurs.

4. There appears to be a *genetic component* in the teratogenic response. Many such effects are species-specific. About 75 percent of the women exposed to thalidomide did not appear to exhibit teratogenic responses to it. It has been suggested that this group may include individuals who lack a genetic background that enhances sensitivity to the drug.

5. The *physiological condition of the mother* may also influence the sensitivity of an embryo to a drug. Very young women and those approaching the menopause appear to be more susceptible than other pregnant women. An inadequate or unbalanced diet may also increase the incidence of birth defects. Maternal diseases such as diabetes mellitus, hypertension, and liver disorders may enhance the potential effects of drugs on the embryo.

Mechanism of teratogenic action. The mechanism of the teratogenic action of drugs is poorly understood. There are three general ways in which drugs may so act:

1. They may have a direct action on the embryo following their passage across the placenta.
2. They may have an indirect action by influencing the accessibility of nutrients to the embryo or fetus. Thus, trypan blue is a potent teratogen that does not cross the placenta but is thought to compromise the activities of enzymes in this membrane.
3. An action on the metabolism of the mother may influence the development of the embryo. In animals hypoglycemic drugs may exert teratogenic effects in this way, though they also can cross the placenta.

The basic mechanism of action is thought to involve such factors as toxic effects on the proliferation of embryonic cells, interactions with DNA, and interference with the processes of genetic transcription and translation resulting in deficiencies of essential nutrients and enzymes. It is also considered possible that some drugs may act directly to disturb the functions of certain enzymes that are involved in embryonic differentiation.

Effects of proven teratogens. Folic acid is an essential growth factor, whose effects certain drugs such as methotrexate and aminopterin (antimetabolite drugs) can antagonize. These *folic acid antagonists* can thus inhibit the growth of cells, and so are used to treat cancer. In rats they result in the resorption of embryos, an observation that led to the testing of aminopterin as an abortifacient drug in women (see Thiersch, 1952). It was administered between the 3rd and 8th week of pregnancy. In some instances, however, the embryos survived, and on examination following later spontaneous or surgical abortions they were seen to exhibit a number of abnormalities, including cleft palate, hydrocephaly, and visceral disorders.

Thalidomide is a nonbarbiturate sedative-hypnotic that was widely used in West Germany and the United Kingdom in the late 1950s. It was considered to be especially "safe" and was taken by pregnant women as a tranquilizer and antiemetic. In 1961 (see below in this chapter, under "The development of new drugs"), it was observed that about 20 percent of the pregnant women who had taken the drug prior to the 8th week after conception gave birth to infants with grossly deformed limbs. The most susceptible period appeared to be from the 20th to the 35th days after conception. The most obvious effects are a general reduction in the size of the limb bones and an absence of digits so that the extremities are markedly shortened (phocomelia = seal-like). Spontaneous abortion and neonatal mortality occurred in many of the fetuses and infants who had been exposed to thalidomide, mostly reflecting other types of abnormalities involving the heart, kidneys, and gut. Many such deformed infants, however, survived.

Drugs with the activity of the female sex hormones progesterone and estrogens have been widely used (in "at risk" pregnancies) in efforts to prevent spontaneous or threatened abortions. Their efficacy for this purpose has, however, never been confirmed, and is currently in serious doubt.

In 1971 (see Herbst et al., 1975) it was observed that many cases of clear-cell adenocarcinoma of the vagina and cervix in young women could be related to the administration of *estrogens*, predominantly diethylstilbestrol or DES, to their mothers during their pregnancy. Exposure to the drug usually occurred prior to the 13th week. DES thus appears to be acting as a teratogenic carcinogen, the latter effect usually not being manifested until about 15 to 20 years later. This discovery has resulted in a widespread screening program of such children.

Progesterone-like preparations (*progestins*) of drugs have also been widely used in attempts to prevent threatened abortions. Some of these, such as ethisterone and norethindrone, have significant male sex hormone (androgen) activity (see Wilkins, 1960) and have been observed to have a virilizing effect on female fetuses. Differentiation of the external genitalia may be male-like and result in pseudohermaphrodism if the drugs are given in the first 3 months of pregnancy. Less dramatic effects, such as an enlargement of the clitoris, may also occur when large doses of such hormone-like preparations are used even later in gestation.

As described earlier in this section, the development of the nervous system may be responsive to the actions of drugs throughout the fetal period. The sex hormones may play a role in this process. It has been reported (Reinisch, 1977) that both the male and female children of mothers who were given estrogens or progestins during pregnancy may exhibit differences from other children in their temperaments and personalities. These interesting observations were made from a series of psychological tests. For instance, it was observed that the progestin "group subjects were significantly more independent, sensitive, individualistic, self-assured and self-sufficient than the offspring of the (estrogen) group, while the (estrogen) group subjects were more group-oriented and group-dependent" (Reinisch, 1977, p. 562).

Monitoring and evaluation of adverse effects of drugs

Serious adverse reactions to drug therapy are not especially frequent, but, as we have seen, they may carry a high risk of morbidity and even result in the death of the patient. Iatrogenic, or drug-induced, disease is a significant problem. It is thus important that information about the toxic and side effects of drugs be recorded and made available, preferably in some digestible form, to physicians. The collection of the data, however, is not always easy, and in the past it has often been many years before a serious toxic side effect has been positively identified. For instance, the abuse of some nonnarcotic analgesic mixtures has been associated with a toxic action on the kidney, in which a necrosis of the renal papilla occurs. This condition often necessitates dialysis procedures or kidney transplants. The effect appears to be mainly related to the presence of phenacetin in such mixtures. This drug was first introduced into medicine in 1886, but its toxic action was not recognized until a few years ago. Phenformin is an oral hypoglycemic drug used in the treatment of mature-onset diabetes mellitus. It was withdrawn from use in the United States in July 1977, nearly 20 years after it was introduced. It was found to carry a risk of precipitating lactic acidosis, a condition that is often fatal. However, such a prolonged time lag in identifying toxic effects of drugs is not inevitable. In May 1979 the uricosuric-diuretic drug ticrynafen was approved for use in the United States. In January 1980 (less than 9 months later) it was withdrawn because it was reported that 52 of about 300,000 patients treated with the drug developed liver damage, which resulted in a number of deaths. It would appear that interest in, and reporting of, toxic effects of drugs may be improving.

It is clearly difficult to collect such information owing to its wide-

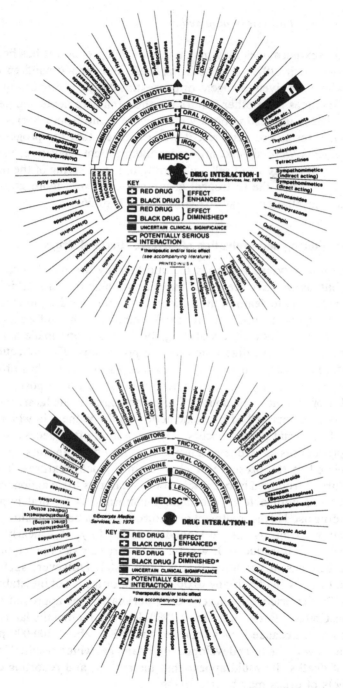

Figure 23. The MEDISC. This simple device can be used to predict possible interactions between drugs that are being given concurrently to the same

spread dispersal, the large numbers of patients who may be involved, and the multiple activities of physicians. Committees and registers are frequently organized in hospitals to monitor such effects, and have been organized at the national level in some countries. Indeed, it is sometimes even illegal, as in Sweden, not to report adverse reactions to drugs. Physicians generally, however, are considered to have a poor record in this respect, especially in the United States, where it has been attributed to the fear of self-incrimination and litigation. Such reports of adverse reactions to drugs may take the form of published letters in journals, or the manufacturer may be notified. In the United Kingdom, the Committee on Safety of Medicine is the main and official recipient of such information, and it periodically issues forms to physicians on which they can record their suspicions. In the United States, The Pharmaceutical Association collects such material and periodically publishes supplements to its compendium *Evaluations of Drug Interactions*. The American Medical Association has a Registry of Adverse Reactions, which also issues bulletins. The FDA collects and collates such material, but its record has been criticized (Marshall, 1980). The World Health Organization has an international register of adverse responses to drugs.

More precisely designed surveys to evaluate adverse reactions and interactions to particular drug preparations, in a general in-hospital situation involving all drugs, are proceeding. In the United States such a program hs been under way since 1966: The Boston Collaborative Surveillance Program (BCDSP). It uses specially trained nurse monitors in a hospital setting, and the results have been periodically published in such journals as *The New England Journal of Medicine*, *The Lancet*, and *JAMA*.

The Stobhill Hospital in Glascow has had a program since 1972 that collates information about drug interactions (Whiting and Goldberg, 1977). The information has been collected and sorted using a simple mechanical system (expensive computers are not always necessary!) of overlaid cardboard discs. This Drug Disc or MEDISC has been printed by the Excerpta Medica Foundation (Figure 23) and provides an inex-

Caption to Fig. 23 (*cont.*)
patient. It was originally devised and prepared by B. Whiting, A. Goldberg, and P. S. Waldie (*Lancet* 1:1037, 1973). It consists of three concentric discs two of which are superimposed on each side. The smaller ones on each side can be rotated in an arc to expose six different types of responses to a particular drug interaction. About 1000 such interactions between about 120 drugs are summarized. (Reproduced with permission of Excerpta Medica Services Inc., Princeton, New Jersey)

pensive, portable, and convenient method for predicting possible interactions between drugs.

Drugs and environmental chemicals

The air we breathe, the water we drink, and the food that we eat are laced with a host of chemical compounds, which may influence the effects of the drugs we take. Some of these compounds are placed there intentionally, as a possible contribution to our good health or for enjoyment. These substances include fluoride in drinking water, additives such as vitamins, minerals, and preservatives in our food, and substances to influence our mood, such as caffeine in tea, ethanol in cocktails, and nicotine in cigarettes. Artificial colors and flavors contribute cosmetic adornment to our diet. Many other types of substances are not intentionally present, and those that may be harmful are called *pollutants*. The latter include carbon monoxide and sulfur dioxide in air, residues of organic compounds and toxic minerals, such as lead, in drinking water, and the remains of livestock feed additives and pesticides in food. There can be considerable geographical variation in such pollution, and some industrial occupations may be especially prone to exposure to certain chemicals. Thus, shipyard workers may be exposed to the potential carcinogenic effects of the asbestos they work with, chemical workers to the hepatotoxic solvents that they decant, pharmaceutical laboratory workers to the actions of the drugs they make, and agricultural workers to the pesticides they use. Accumulation of such toxic substances may occur through the lungs, gut, and skin.

Interactions of environmental chemicals with drugs

Direct interactions. Chemicals and drugs may have a direct, additive or inhibitory, effect. *Caffeine* belongs to a group of drugs called the xanthines. This group of chemicals occurs as plant alkaloids and includes theophylline and theobromine. They can stimulate the central nervous system, and so prevent sleep, and can even antagonize the effects of hypnotic drugs (sleeping pills) such as the barbiturates. They can also relax certain types of smooth muscle, including the bronchi, and so can be useful drugs in attacks of asthma. Caffeine and its relatives also stimulate the heart, where they can potentiate the effects of epinephrine. We enjoy the effects of caffeine on the central nervous system when we drink tea, coffee, and cola drinks. Its actions, however, can antagonize the effects of hypnotic and sedative drugs that we may take to help us sleep. Caffeine's action on the heart may even result in irregularities in its beat. The taking of large amounts of coffee may thus be counter to the intended actions of drugs we may take in heart disease, such as antiarrythmic and antianginal agents. Caffeine can also stimulate the secretion of gastric juices, which may be undesirable in peptic ulcer disease.

Smoking *tobacco* is probably the most common example of drug abuse. Its principal active ingredient is nicotine, which contributes to its popularity. Nicotine can stimulate the central nervous system and in excess can even result in tremor and convulsions. In confirmed smokers it produces an increase in the heart rate and a small increase in the blood pressure. These effects are mainly the result of the stimulation of sympathetic ganglia and the release of epinephrine from the adrenal medulla. The cardiovascular effects of smoking may also be unfavorable in patients being treated with drugs for heart disease. An important interaction is seen in women who use oral contraceptives. Habitual smokers over the age of 30 years who also take oral contraceptive pills have an increased risk of dying from cardiovascular disorders (see Kuenssberg et al., 1977; editorial, 1977).

Some natural foods including plants of the Brassica family (e.g., cabbage, kale, and Swedish turnips) contain chemical compounds (thiocyanates and L-5-vinyl-2-thiooxyzolidine or goitrin) that can block the ability of the thyroid gland to produce its hormones (see Clements, 1960). Such chemicals can produce a compensatory enlargement of the thyroid gland called goiter. This disorder commonly occurs in certain geographic areas where a deficiency of iodine exists in the soil, as iodine is an essential constituent of the thyroid hormones. In 1949 many schoolchildren in Tasmania (see Clements, 1955) were found to be goitrous, and they were given a weekly supplement of iodine in the form of a 10-mg tablet of potassium iodide. A survey made in 1954 showed that although the incidence of goiter had declined in the older children, there appeared to be a resurgence of the disorder in younger children. Another factor, which was complicating the picture, seemed to have appeared in the interim period. A free milk scheme for the children had been started during this time, and in order to meet the additional demand for milk some dairy farmers fed their cows on thousand-headed kale, a member of the Brassica family. The milk of these cows was found to contain antithyroid substances, which were antagonizing the effects of the potassium iodide supplements.

Indirect interactions. Environmental chemicals and drugs may interact indirectly. Hydrocarbon compounds, in *cigarette smoke,* and pesticides can induce the formation of liver enzymes, and so may increase the rate of metabolism of drugs. Some *insecticides* are inhibitors of cholinesterase. Examples include tetraethylpyrophosphate (TEPP), malathion, and parathion. Illness and death have resulted from the ingestion of these chemicals, and as a result of occupational exposure to them. The effects may be cumulative so that serum cholinesterase levels may decline to low levels. This enzyme mediates the inactivation of a number of natural compounds and drugs, including some local anesthetics, such as procaine, and the muscular relaxant drug succinylcholine. The latter's effect is normally brief, owing to its rapid inactivation. However, patients who have low cholinesterase levels resulting from exposure to such pesticides, may have prolonged responses to such drugs.

Food–drug interactions. Some substances in our diet may interact unfavorably with the drugs we take. Probably the most dramatic example involves antidepressant drugs such as phenelzine and nialamide, which inhibit the tissue enzyme monoamine oxidase (MAO). This enzyme plays a major role in the inactivation of the endogenous amines epinephrine and norepinephrine. It also can destroy exogenous amines such as tyramine. This amino acid is present in high concentrations in certain foods, such as some cheeses and wines. Patients who are being treated with MAO oxidase inhibitor drugs are advised to avoid such delicacies because the tyramine present then accumulates at excessive levels in the body and initiates a release of norepinephrine, which is also present at higher than normal levels in nerve terminals. The blood pressure thus rises, an effect that can be disastrous and has resulted in deaths from cerebral hemorrhage. A toxicologically alert playwright wrote a murder mystery, which was performed by the British Broadcasting Corporation, in which this drug interaction played a central, fatal, role.

Inadvertent contamination. Contamination by drugs may occur inadvertently from the environment in rather unexpected ways. Workers in pharmaceutical factories may accumulate and respond to the drugs that they are making. This is a special danger if the drugs can be absorbed through the skin or inhaled. A recent example involved an inhibition of adrenocortical function in workers making *corticosteroid* *hormone* preparations. These drugs, in low concentrations, can inhibit the release of corticotropin from the pituitary gland, and this lack results in a depression of cortisol secretion from the adrenal cortex. The effect is reversible, but it may take many months before normal activity is restored.

Diethylstilbestrol (DES) has been widely used in the meat industry to improve the quality and foster a more efficient weight gain in cattle, sheep, and chickens. In chickens, pellets may be implanted in the neck just below the head, whereas in cattle they are placed at the base of the ear. It is important that these parts of the animal be discarded following slaughtering. A more widely used procedure is the addition of diethylstilbestrol to the feed of steers. This improves the efficiency of the conversion of their food intake to meat, and there is an increased weight gain of 10 to 25 percent. The mechanism appears to involve an anabolic effect. Such feed is withdrawn from the animals at least 48 hours prior to slaughtering, when the levels of the drug are usually undetectable in most edible tissues. However, DES has been found in some instances, at greater than acceptable levels, in the liver. Public discomfort about the possible carcinogenic effects of such residues of estrogens led to the banning of this practice in many countries, including the United Kingdom, Canada, Australia, West Germany, and the United States.

Topical *corticosteroid preparations* are widely used in the treatment of skin diseases. Two instances were recently described (Stankler and Bewsher, 1978) in which such steroids were transferred during sexual intercourse from the genital region of a husband to his wife. Corticosteroids reduce resistance to infection, and the contamination of the wife resulted in the proliferation of a vaginal candidal infection.

The development of new drugs

Identification

The identification of compounds that may be used as drugs, with properties effective in the treatment of a disease, involves the utilization of tissue culture techniques and live animals and clinical testing on human subjects (see Johnson and Johnson, 1977). This process may extend over many years. Drug companies often screen several thousand compounds a year in such a search. The list may be narrowed down, as a result, to less than a dozen putative drugs, which are considered worthy of more extensive investigation. Of these maybe only one or two, or even none at all, will eventually be marketed. It is considered that the successful introduction of one new drug every 2 to 3 years constitutes a success rate sufficient to justify such research programs. A fascinating autobiographical account, *Discovery, Development and Delivery of New Drugs*, has been written by Dr. K. H. Beyer (1978), dealing with such research programs.

A putative or candidate drug, once identified, goes through two further stages of development, the preclinical and clinical phases, which take an average of 8 years, though the time required can be less than that.

Preclinical phase

Development of manufacturing process. The development of a suitable manufacturing process that assures adequate supplies of the drug, at a not excessive cost, while assuring the purity and stability of the compound is an essential first step.

Development of analytical methods. Analytical methods need to be devised so that the levels of the drug in the body tissues and fluids can be readily measured. Radiolabelled forms of the drug may be made that will facilitate its future study.

Studies of drug fate. Studies, using animals, to define the fate, including the *distribution, metabolism,* and *excretion* of the drug in the body, are undertaken. These investigations may involve measurements, over various periods of time after administration of the drug, of its concentrations in the tissues and blood. Losses in the urine, bile, and feces are also monitored. It is desirable to identify the metabolites of the drug. The effectiveness on blood and tissue levels of different routes of administration are compared. If radiolabelled preparations of the drug are available, then such studies may be considerably simplified, and autoradiographic methods may even be used to see where the drug goes in the body. The identification of its metabolites may also be facilitated by such isotopic preparations of the drug.

Toxicity studies. Toxicity studies are performed on animals of both sexes. Usually two rodents (such as rats and mice) and one nonrodent (e.g., rabbits, but dogs and monkeys are more expensive alternatives) are used.

The *lethal dose* (LD_{50} and LD_{100}) is determined in acute toxicity studies in which the dose is progressively increased. Oral and intravenous routes of administration are used. The responses of the animals, the causes of death, and the terminal blood and tissue concentrations of the drug are observed. When the maximum tolerated dose is known, it is maintained for several weeks so that any effects on tissue pathology can be observed.

Chronic toxicity is tested using a range of sublethal doses, which are initially administered for a period of about 6 months. Subsequently, however, this period is extended to the lifetime of the animal. If possible the highest doses in these chronic toxicity studies should be about 10 times the effective therapeutic dose in man. Various parameters, such as food intake, blood chemistry and pathology, and blood pressure, are routinely monitored. At the end of this initial period of the chronic-toxicity tests some of the animals are killed, and their tissue pathology is investigated. In some of the remaining animals the drug is withdrawn, so that it can be ascertained at a later date if any identified pathological changes are reversible.

Possible *teratogenic* effects on the fetus are investigated following administration of the drug to pregnant animals, usually rats and rabbits.

Effects on *fertility* are performed on male and female animals, usually rats. These studies are carried out over three generations.

Tests for *mutagenic effects* of the drugs may also be performed by cytological examination on the germ cells of these animals and in cultures of microorganisms.

Carcinogenicity is monitored by observing the incidence of malignant and benign tumors.

On the basis of all these observations on animals a clinical trial in man may be deemed feasible, and possibly rewarding.

Clinical phase

Until about 20 years ago the introduction of new drugs and the use of old drugs in clinical practice was largely at the discretion of apothecaries, pharmacists, pharmaceutical manufacturing companies, and individual physicians. Indeed it is doubtful if many of the drugs in regular use in the early part of this century would gain the license of registration that is now necessary to market a drug in most countries. Many such old drugs are still currently available, often despite a doubtful efficacy. Such drugs are, however, undergoing critical review in some countries, including the United States and the United Kingdom; but the process will take a long time to complete. When a toxic action or serious side effect does become apparent, legal devices usually exist for withdrawing the drug from clinical use. The drug companies are usually fully cooperative in such matters, but controversies do occur. Recent examples of such reevaluations include restriction in the use of the analgesic phenacetin, which has a renal toxicity in some circumstances, and the orally active antidiabetic drug phenformin, which may precipitate lactic acidosis. Such clinical observations have led to restrictions in the use, and even the withdrawal, of such drugs in some countries. National regulations to control the clinical testing and use of drugs have followed in the wake of a series of therapeutic disasters.

In 1937 in the United States the use of a preparation of the newly developed sulfonamide drugs called elixir of sulfanilamide resulted in at least 73 deaths. This toxicity was due not to the drug itself but the solvent, diethylene glycol, in which it was marketed. This disaster resulted in a congressional investigation and led to the forming of the Food and Drug Administration (FDA). This federal organization oversees the introduction of new drugs and the continued use of old ones.

In 1956 in West Germany and 1958 in the United Kingdom and some British Commonwealth countries, a nonbarbiturate sedative-hypnotic drug called thalidomide (Contergan, Distaval) was introduced into clinical practice. Unfortunately it was widely used by pregnant women. (See earlier in this chapter, under "Teratogenic effects of drugs.") As a result of the observations of some alert physicians in West Germany (Lenz, 1962) and Australia (McBride, 1961) it was noted that there was a marked increase in births of infants who suffered from grossly deformed limbs (phocomelia) (see Figure 24). These children were invariably found to have been born to mothers who had been given thalidomide in early pregnancy. In a survey of several West German obstetrical clinics this condition was found to be virtually unknown prior to 1959, but 10 cases were reported that year and in 1961 the number had risen to 477. Altogether in West Germany about 6000 live births of children occurred with such deformities, and in the United

Figure 24. The first published warnings of the thalidomide "disaster." (Top, from *Lancet 2:*1358, 1961; bottom, from *Lancet 1:*45, 1962)

THALIDOMIDE AND CONGENITAL ABNORMALITIES

SIR,—Congenital abnormalities are present in approximately 1·5% of babies. In recent months I have observed that the incidence of multiple severe abnormalities in babies delivered of women who were given the drug thalidomide ('Distaval') during pregnancy, as an anti-emetic or as a sedative, to be almost 20%.

These abnormalities are present in structures developed from mesenchyme—i.e., the bones and musculature of the gut. Bony development seems to be affected in a very striking manner, resulting in polydactyly, syndactyly, and failure of development of long bones (abnormally short femora and radii).

Have any of your readers seen similar abnormalities in babies delivered of women who have taken this drug during pregnancy?

Hurstville, New South Wales.   W. G. McBRIDE.

₊ In our issue of Dec. 2 we included a statement from the Distillers Company (Biochemicals) Ltd. referring to " reports from two overseas sources possibly associating thalidomide ('Distaval') with harmful effects on the fœtus in early pregnancy ". Pending further investigation, the company decided to withdraw from the market all its preparations containing thalidomide.—ED.L.

THALIDOMIDE AND CONGENITAL ABNORMALITIES

SIR,—Dr. McBride (Dec. 16) describes congenital abnormalities in babies delivered of women who have taken thalidomide. I have seen 52 malformed infants whose mothers had taken ' Contergan ' in early pregnancy, and I understand that contergan is a synonym of thalidomide, others being ' Distaral,' ' Softenon ', ' Neurosedyn ', ' Isomin ', ' Kedavon ', ' Telargan ', and ' Sedalis '.

Since I discussed the possible ætiological role of contergan in human malformations at a conference on Nov. 18, 1961, I have received letters from many places in the German Federal Republic, as well as from Belgium, England, and Sweden, reporting 115 additional cases in which this drug was thought to be the cause.

Though these malformations. . .

Judging from case histories of more than 300 women who have borne normal infants, and of whom none had taken contergan between the 4th and the 8th week after conception, the risk to a fœtus of a mother taking contergan during this period may be definitely higher than 20%. I venture the estimate that at least 2000, possibly more than 3000, " contergan " babies have been born in Western Germany since 1959.

Universitäts-Kinderklinik,
Hamburg-Eppendorf, Germany.   W. LENZ.

Kingdom there were about 500. The drug had not been approved for use in the United States, a fact that has been used in hindsight to justify the wisdom of the FDA regulations. This catastrophe led to the introduction of a statutory law in the United Kingdom that controls the testing, introduction, and use of new drugs. The Safety of Drugs Committee was formed (the Dunlop Committee), which made its initial report in 1963. The Medicines Act became law in 1968. Under this statute there are three bodies concerned with regulating the use of therapeutic drugs in the United Kingdom:

1. The licensing of a drug and the performance of clinical trials is under the control of the ministers of health and agriculture. The actual administration and issuance of the licenses is by the Department of Health and Social Security.
2. The Medicine Commission advises the ministers and if necessary acts as an arbiter between the applicant and the Committee on Safety of Medicines.
3. The Committee on Safety of Medicines (which succeeded the Dunlop Commitee) and its subcommittees initially consider and make recommendations regarding clinical trials and the issuing of licenses to market a drug.

In the United States notice of a proposed clinical trial ("Claimed Investigational Exemption for a New Drug"; the form is called IND) must be filed with the Bureau of Drugs of the FDA, who may object to it within 30 days. In most countries comparable regulations exist, though their stringency varies, and they are not always under governmental control.

Detailed records, often involving individual patients, are usually ultimately required. The results are continually monitored during the progress of the trial. If serious adverse reactions occur, the trial may be stopped.

Expensive and time-wasting duplication of clinical trials on new drugs is often carried out in different countries, where the detailed legal requirements may differ. Attempts are being made, such as in the European Economic Community (EEC), to standardize such requirements. The acceptance in one country, as evidence of safety and efficacy, of clinical trials performed in foreign countries is being pursued and has gained limited, but useful, approval in the United States.

Phase I of the clinical trial involves determination of the drug's safety and toxicity in man. It usually involves an investigation on a small group of people. The choice and availability of human individuals for these studies poses some ethical, legal, and practical problems. Children (except in typical childhood diseases), pregnant and potentially pregnant women, and old people are usually excluded. The terminally ill are not considered to be suitable, as their condition may complicate the results. Volunteers are collected from such groups as prisoners (a formerly very useful source in the United States), students, patients suffering from unrelated diseases, or persons with a resistant form of the disease for which the drug is intended. Financial compensation is often proffered, but other rewards are not, as they may be taken to constitute a bribe or an unethical inducement. The main aim of the Phase I trials is to see what dosages of the drug can be tolerated in man. Small initial doses are progressively increased until putative therapeutic levels are attained, or adverse reactions make further increases in dose intolerable or dangerous.

Phase II trials are aimed at determining the therapeutic efficacy and common side effects of the drug. Usually they involve larger groups than in Phase I, but fewer than 1000 patients, who it is hoped will also benefit from the new drug. The aims are (1) to show that the drug is clinically effective, (2) to define the dose range for its efficacy, and (3) to observe what side effects and adverse reactions may occur and to estimate their frequency.

An appropriate experimental design to allow an objective assessment, based on a statistical analysis of the results, is important, especially as the results of such studies can be quite complex and may be controversial.

Phase III trials are more extensive versions of Phase II and allow for a more detailed analysis of possible side effects, drug interactions, prolonged administration, and, where appropriate, use in children and the elderly. These studies are carried out provided that the results of Phase II are satisfactory, and no objectionable adverse effects have since been observed in the concurrent long-term toxicity trials on animals.

Finally all the information and data are assembled for submission as an application for permission to market the drug. This procedure can involve enormous amounts of paper work, which in the United States is said to average several meters in height. Processing may take from 6 months to as long as 3 years.

Even following the authorized marketing of a drug, patients' responses to it are still monitored, and indeed there was a recent instance in which a drug was subsequently withdrawn. (As described earlier in

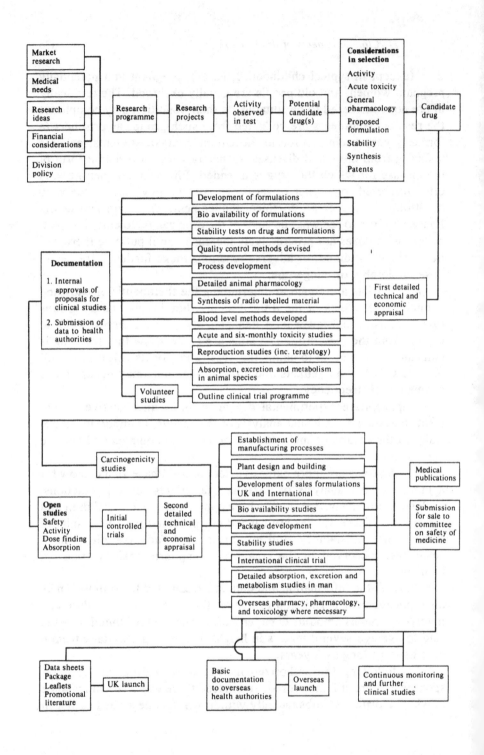

this chapter, under "Monitoring and evaluation of adverse effects of drugs," the uricosuric-diuretic drug ticrynafen – Selacryn – was marketed in May 1979 but withdrawn in January 1980.)

A flow sheet showing the stages in the development of a drug, in this instance from the ICI Company in the United Kingdom, is presented in Figure 25.

Figure 25. Stages in the development of a drug for clinical use, from its discovery to its approval for marketing. This example is from the United Kingdom and was prepared by ICI Ltd., Macclesfield. (From *Birth of a Drug*, ICI Ltd.)

12
Conclusion

Pharmacology is an exact science that rests on a foundation of chemistry, physics, and physiology. It, however, freely borrows its techniques and methods from other scientific disciplines as they are developed. It could, in this respect, be considered parasitic, but as it also donates information, its relationship to other sciences can be considered symbiotic. Probably more than any other such subject it has pure and applied aspects that cannot be disentangled from each other. Drugs have no reality in the absence of their use by man.

Drugs are necessary, and can be evil. Their indiscriminate and nontherapeutic use is usually to be abhored and avoided, and the real necessity for administering them requires circumspection. When they are appropriately used, however, drugs can extend life and alleviate pain and suffering. Many drugs are today quite freely and legally available to the public, both over the counter (OTC) and by medical prescription. They can, however, also be obtained covertly and illicitly. Their proper use in modern society is not only dependent on properly trained physicians but also on an educated public. It is inexcusable for the medical practitioner to fail in his or her role, but one cannot expect universal pharmacological introspection among the public. Attempts to increase the knowledge of people in drug-related matters are being made with the cooperation of the popular press, the pharmaceutical companies, and private and governmental medical organizations. Maybe this subject should be dubbed "social pharmacology" or "community pharmacology." Failure to so inform and educate the public needs to be compensated for by protective legal restrictions on the availability of and accessibility to illicit sources of drugs. A continuing assessment of the alleged benefits and possible dangers of over-the-counter remedies and newly developed drugs is an important contemporary activity of government that does not always receive the moral, and other, support it merits and needs. We have in this century been through the era of the discovery and introduction of many "wonder drugs," and the end is certainly not in sight; but today we tend to tread more carefully. The function of pharmacology is to provide a rational approach to the development and use of such drugs.

References

Albuquerque, E., Daly, J. W., and Witkop, B. 1971. Batrachotoxin: chemistry and pharmacology. *Science 172:*995–1002.

Ames, B. N. 1979. Identifying environmental chemicals causing mutations and cancer. *Science 204:*587–93.

Ariëns, E. J. 1966. Molecular pharmacology, a basis for drug design. *Prog. Drug Res. 10:*429–529.

1979. Receptors: from fiction to fact. *TIPS 1:*11–15.

Ariëns, E. J., and Simonis, A. M. 1964a. A molecular basis for drug action. *J. Pharm. Pharmacol. 16:*137–57.

1964b. A molecular basis for drug action. The interaction of one or more drugs with different receptors. *J. Pharm. Pharmacol. 16:*289–312.

Beckett, A. H., and Casy, A. F. 1954. Synthetic analgesics: stereochemical considerations. *J. Pharm. Pharmacol. 6:*986–99.

1965. Analgesics and their antagonists: biochemical aspects and structure activity relationships. *Prog. Med. Chem. 4:*171–218.

Bergeron, J. J. M., Levine, G., Sikstrom, R., O'Shaughnessy, D., Kopriwa, B., Nadler, N. J., and Posner, B. I. 1977. Polypeptide hormone binding sites in vivo: initial localization of ^{125}I-insulin to hepatocyte plasmalemma as visualized by electron microscope radioautography. *Proc. Natl. Acad. Sci. U.S.A. 74:*5051–5.

Beyer, K. H. 1978. *Discovery, Development and Delivery of New Drugs*. New York: Spectrum.

Catt, K. J., and Dufau, M. L. 1977. Peptide hormone receptors. *Annu. Rev. Physiol. 39:*529–57.

Catt, K. J., Harwood, J. P., Aguilera, G., and Dufau, M. L. 1979. Hormonal regulation of peptide receptors and target cell responses. *Nature (Lond.) 280:*109–16.

Chan, L., and O'Malley, B. W. 1976. Mechanism of action of sex steroid hormones (part 1). *N. Engl. J. Med. 294:*1322–8.

Changeux, J-P., Thiéry, J., Tung, Y., and Kittel, C. 1967. On the cooperativity of biological membranes. *Proc. Natl. Acad. Sci. U.S.A. 57:*335–41.

Clark, C. A., Evans, D. A. P., Harris, R., McConnell, R. B., and Woodrow, J. C. 1968. Genetics in medicine: a review. 2. Pharmacogenetics. *Quart. J. Med. 37:*183–219.

Clegg, D. J. 1971. Teratology. *Annu. Rev. Pharmacol. 11:*409–24.

Clements, F. W. 1955. A thyroid blocking agent as a cause of endemic goitre in Tasmania: preliminary communication. *Med. J. Aust. 42(2):*369–71.
1960. Naturally occurring goitrogens. *Br. Med. Bull. 16:*133–7.
Clouet, D. H., and Iwatsubo, K. 1975. Mechanisms of tolerance to and dependence on narcotic analgesic drugs. *Annu. Rev. Pharmacol. Toxicol. 15:*49–71.
Collier, H. O. J. 1980. Cellular site of opiate dependence. *Nature (Lond.) 283:*625–9.
Cuatrecasas, P., Hollenberg, M. D., Chang, K-J., and Bennett, V. 1975. Hormone receptor complexes and their modulation of membrane function. *Rec. Prog. Horm. Res. 31:*37–84.
De Meyts, P., Bianco, A. R., and Roth, J. 1976. Site–site interactions among insulin receptors. Characterization of the negative cooperativity. *J. Biol. Chem. 251:*1877–88.
Editorial. 1972. The bioavailability of digoxin. *Lancet 1:*311–12.
Editorial. 1977. Mortality associated with the Pill. *Lancet 2:*747–8.
Fraumeni, J. F. 1979. Epidemiological studies of cancer. In *Carcinogens: Identification and Mechanisms,* ed. by A. C. Griffin and C. R. Shaw, pp. 51–63. New York: Raven Press.
Freychet, P., Roth, J., and Neville, D. M. 1971. Insulin receptors in the liver: specific binding of [^{125}I]insulin to the plasma membrane and its relation to insulin bioactivity. *Proc. Natl. Acad. Sci. U.S.A. 68:*1833–7.
Furchgott, R. F. 1978. Pharmacological characterization of receptors: its relation to radioligand-binding studies. *Fed. Proc. 37:*115–20.
Goldberg, L. (ed.) 1973. *Carcinogenesis Testing of Chemicals.* Cleveland, Ohio: CRC Press.
Goldstein, J. L., Anderson, R. G. W., and Brown, M. S. 1979. Coated pits, coated vesicles, and receptor-mediated endocytosis. *Nature (Lond.) 279:*679–85.
Gorden, P., Carpentier, J-L., Freychet, P., LeCam, A., and Orci, L. 1978. Intracellular translocation of iodine-125-labeled insulin: direct demonstration in isolated hepatocytes. *Science 200:*782–5.
Grasso, A., Alema, S., Rufini, S., and Senni, M. I. 1980. Black widow spider toxin-induced calcium fluxes and transmitter release in a neurosecretory cell line. *Nature (Lond.) 283:*774–6.
Greaves, M. F. 1977. Membrane receptor–adenylate cyclase relationships. *Nature (Lond.) 265:*681–3.
Greenblatt, D. J., and Koch-Weser, J. 1975a. Clinical pharmacokinetics (part 1). *N. Engl. J. Med. 293:*702–5.
1975b. Clinical pharmacokinetics. (part 2). *N. Engl. J. Med. 293:*964–70.
Gund, P., Andose, J. D., Rhodes, J. B., and Smith, G. M. 1980. Three-dimensional molecular modeling and drug design. *Science 208:*1425–31.
Herbst, A. L., Poskanzer, D. C., Robboy, S. J., Friedlander, L., and Scully, R. E. 1975. Prenatal exposure to stilbestrol. A prospective comparison of exposed female offspring with unexposed controls. *N. Engl. J. Med. 292:*334–9.

Herington, A. D., Veith, N., and Burger, H. G. 1976. Characterization of the binding of human growth hormone to microsomal membranes from rat liver. *Biochem. J. 158:*61–9.

Hollenberg, M. D., and Cuatrecasas, P. 1978. Membrane receptors and hormone action: recent developments. *Prog. Neuro-Psychopharmacol. 2:*287–302.

Jard, S., and Bockaert, J. (1975). Stimulus–response coupling in neurohypophysial peptide target cells. *Physiol. Rev. 55:*489–536.

Johnson, F. N., and Johnson, S. (eds.) 1977. *Clinical Trials.* Oxford: Blackwell.

Kalow, W. 1962. *Pharmacogenetics, Heredity and the Response to Drugs.* Philadelphia: Saunders

Karlin, A. 1967. On the application of "a plausible model" of allosteric proteins to the receptor for acetylcholine. *J. Theor. Biol. 16:*306–20.

Koch-Weser, J. 1974a. Bioavailability of drugs (part 1). *N. Engl. J. Med. 291:*233–7.

1974b. Bioavailability of drugs (part 2). *N. Engl. J. Med. 291:*503–6.

Koch-Weser, J., and Sellers, E. M. 1976a. Binding of drugs to serum albumin (part 1). *N. Engl. J. Med. 294:*311–16.

1976b. Binding of drugs to serum albumin (part 2). *N. Engl. J. Med. 294:*526–31.

Kolata, G. B. 1978. Polypeptide hormones: what are they doing in cells? *Science 201:*895–7.

Kuenssberg, E. V., Kay, C. R., Dewhurst, J., and Booth, R. J. 1977. Recommendations from the findings by the RCGP oral contraceptive study on the mortality risks of oral contraceptive users. *Br. Med. J. 2:*947.

Lefkowitz, F. J. 1976. β-Adrenergic receptors: recognition and regulation. *N. Engl. J. Med. 295:*323–8.

Lenz, W. 1962. Thalidomide and congenital abnormalities. *Lancet 1:*45.

Lindenbaum, J., Mellow, M. H., Blackstone, M. O., and Butler, V. P. 1971. Variation in biological availability of digoxin from four preparations. *N. Engl. J. Med. 285:*1344–7.

Lodish, H. F., and Rothman, J. E. 1979. The assembly of cell membranes. *Sci. Am. 240:*48–63.

McBride, W. G. 1961. Thalidomide and congenital abnormalities. *Lancet 2:*1358.

Maguire, M. E., Ross, E. M., and Gilman, A. G. 1977. β-Adrenergic receptor: ligand binding properties and interaction with adenyl cyclase. In *Advances in Nucleotide Research,* vol. 8, ed. by P. Greegard and G. A. Robison, pp. 1–83. New York: Raven Press.

Manninen, V., Melin, J., and Härtel, G. 1971. Serum digoxin concentrations during treatment with different preparations. *Lancet 2:*934–5.

Marshall, E. 1980. A prescription for monitoring drugs. *Science 207:*853–955.

O'Malley, B. W., and Schrader, W. T. 1976. The receptors of steroid hormones. *Sci. Am. 234:*32–43.

Paton, W. D. M. 1961. A theory of drug action based on the rate of drug–receptor combination. *Proc. R. Soc. Lond. B 154:*21–69.

Pickup, J. C., Keen, H., Parsons, J. A., Alberti, K. G. M. M., and Rowe, A. S. 1979. Continuous subcutaneous insulin infusion: improved blood-glucose and intermediary-metabolite control in diabetics. *Lancet 1:*1255–8.

Propping, P. 1978. Pharmacogenetics. *Rev. Physiol. Biochem. Pharmacol. 83:*123–73.

Rang, H. P. 1971. Drug receptors and their function. *Nature (Lond.) 231:*91–6.

Reinisch, J. M. 1977. Prenatal exposure of human foetuses to synthetic progestin and oestrogen affects personality. *Nature (Lond.) 266:*561–2.

Roth, J., Kahn, C. R., Lesniak, M. A., Gorden, P., De Meyts, P., Megyesi, K., Neville, D. M., Gavin, J. R., Soll, A. H., Freychet, P., Goldfine, I. D., Bar, R. S., and Archer, J. A. 1975. Receptors for insulin NSILA-s, and growth hormone: application to disease states in man. *Rec. Prog. Horm. Res. 31:*95–126.

Scatchard, G. 1949. The attractions of proteins for small molecules and ions. *Ann. N.Y. Acad. Sci. 51:*660–72.

Schild, H. O. 1957. Drug antagonism and pA_x. *Pharmacol Rev. 9:*242–6.

Schrader, W. T., and O'Malley, B. W. 1978. *Laboratory Methods Manual for Hormone Action and Molecular Endocrinology 1978.* Houston: Houston Biological Associates.

Schueler, F. W. 1960. *Chemodynamics and Drug Design,* pp. 140–98. New York: McGraw-Hill.

Sclessinger, J., Schechter, Y., Willingham, M. C., and Pastan, I. 1978. Direct visualization of binding, aggregation, and internalization of insulin and epidermal growth factor in living fibroblast cells. *Proc. Natl. Acad. Sci. U.S.A. 75:*2659–63.

Sharma, S., Klee, W. A., and Nirenberg, M. 1975. Dual regulation of adenylate cyclase accounts for narcotic dependence and tolerance. *Proc. Natl. Acad. Sci. U.S.A. 72:*3092–6.

   1977. Opiate-dependent modulation of adenylate cyclase. *Proc. Natl. Acad. Sci. U.S.A. 74:*3365–9.

Sharp, G. W. G., Komack, C. L., and Leaf, A. 1966. Studies on the binding of aldosterone in the toad bladder. *J. Clin. Invest. 45:*450–9.

Snyder, S. H. 1977. Opiate receptors and internal opiates. *Sci. Am. 236:*44–56.

Stankler, L., and Bewsher, P. D. 1978. Adverse reaction to a topical steroid transferred by physical contact. *Br. Med. J. 2:*399–400.

Thiersch, J. B. 1952. Therapeutic abortions with a folic acid antagonist, 4-aminopteroylglutamic acid (4-amino P.G.A.) administered by the oral route. *Am. J. Obstet. Gynecol. 63:*1298–1304.

Thron, C. D. 1973. On the analysis of pharmacological experiments in terms of allosteric receptor model. *Mol. Pharmacol. 9:*1–9.

Tuchmann-Duplessis, H. 1975. *Drug Effects on the Fetus.* Sydney: ADIS Press.

Urry, D. W., and Walter, R. 1971. Proposed conformation of oxytocin in solution. *Proc. Natl. Acad. Sci. U.S.A. 68:*956–8.

Walter, R. 1977. Identification of sites in oxytocin involved in uterine receptor recognition and activation. *Fed. Proc. 36:*1872–8.

Walter, R., Smith, C. W., Mehta, P. K., Boonjarern, S., Arruda, J. A. L., and

Kurtzman, N. A. 1977. Conformational consideration of vasopressin as a guide to development of biological probes and therapeutic agents. In *Disturbances in Body Fluid Osmolality,* ed. by T. E. Andreoli, J. J. Grantham, and F. C. Rector, pp. 1–36. Bethesda, Md.: American Physiological Society.

Weisburger, E. K. 1978. Mechanisms of chemical carcinogenesis. *Annu. Rev. Pharmacol. Toxicol. 18:*395–415.

Whiting, B., and Goldberg, A. 1977. The use of the drug disc (MEDISC): a warning system for drug interactions. In *Drug Interactions,* ed. by D. G. Graham-Smith, pp. 21–31. Baltimore, Md.: University Park Press.

Whiting, B., Goldberg, A. and Waldie, P. S. 1973. The drug disc: warning system for drug interactions. *Lancet 1:* 1037.

Wilkins, L. 1960. Masculinization of female fetus due to use of orally given progestins. *J.A.M.A. 172:* 1028–32.

Wilson, J. G. 1974. Factors determining the teratogenicity of drugs. *Annu. Rev. Pharmacol. 14:* 205–17.

Glossary of drugs named in the text

acetaminophen: nonnarcotic analgesic, antipyretic; can result in necrosis of liver in toxic doses.

acetanilid: nonnarcotic analgesic, related to acetaminophen. Not in current use.

acetazolamide: weak diuretic; inhibits carbonic anhydrase. Now mostly used for treatment of glaucoma.

acetylsalicyclic acid: see *aspirin*.

ACTH: see *corticotropin*.

actinomycin D: antibiotic; inhibits RNA depolymerase and genetic transcription (nucleus). Used in cancer chemotherapy.

ADH: antidiuretic hormone. See *vasopressin*.

aldosterone: steroid hormone from adrenal cortex. Produces urinary Na retention and K loss. Not used therapeutically.

allopurinol: blocks formation of uric acid; xanthine oxidase inhibitor. Used in treatment of gout.

aluminum hydroxide: gastric antacid; binds phosphate in gut. Used in treatment of dyspepsia, peptic ulcer, and to limit phosphate absorption in association renal dialysis.

amiloride: potassium-sparing diuretic, with weak diuretic action; reduces K excretion (not used in United States).

aminopterin: "antimetabolite drug." Used in cancer chemotherapy; has teratogenic action.

aminopyrine: nonnarcotic analgesic. The occurrence of agranulocytosis has led to its disuse.

amitryptyline: tricyclic antidepressant.

amphetamine: sympathomimetic; stimulates central nervous system; suppresses appetite but not recommended for such use.

amphotericin B: polyene antifungal drug; has nephrotoxic side effects.

androgenic steroids: testosterone (male sex hormone)-like; produced by testes, adrenal cortex.

anticoagulants: prevent blood clotting. Heparin, dicumarol, warfarin.

anticonvulsants: used to treat epilepsy and other convulsive disorders. Phenobarbital, phenytoin, diazepam (Valium), primidone, carbamazepine.

antihistamines: histamine H_1-antagonists, diphenhydramine, promethazine, cyclizine, etc. used for motion sickness, allergies, hypnotics (H_2-receptor antagonist = cimetidine for peptic ulcer).

aspirin: salicylate, nonnarcotic analgesic; antiinflammatory in rheumatoid fever, rheumatoid arthritis; reduces body temperature in fever.

atropine: plant alkaloid; anticholinergic premedication for anesthesia, diarrhea, and to dilate pupils. Blocks parasympathetic muscarinic effects of acetylcholine.

A23187: carboxylic acid, Ca ionophore; increases Ca exchanges across cell membrane (not used therapeutically).

batrachotoxin: steroidal alkaloid from skin of a Colombian frog. Increases Na permeability of nerve and muscle.

beclomethasone: inhalable corticosteroid. Used in treatment of asthma.

belladona: plant alkaloid. See *atropine* for actions.

bishydroxycoumarin: oral anticoagulant.

caffeine: xanthine alkaloid; stimulant in coffee and tea.

calcium carbonate: gastric antacid. Used as "filler" in pharmaceutical preparations.

carbamazepine: anticonvulsant. Used in treatment of epilepsy.

carbutamide: early oral hypoglycemic drug. Incidence of agranulocytosis has led to its disuse.

cardiac glycosides: digitalis, digoxin, digitoxin, ouabain. Used in treatment of congestive heart failure and cardiac arrhythmias. Increase force of contraction of heart muscle; inhibit enzyme Na-K activated ATPase.

chloral hydrate: hypnotic and sedative drug.

chloramphenicol: antibiotic; can result in aplastic anemia.

chlordiazepoxide (librium): benzodiazepine. Used as tranquilizer and in alcohol withdrawal syndrome.

chlorothiazide: diuretic drug. Used in treatment of edema (congestive heart failure), hypertension, nephrogenic diabetes insipidus. Side effects include loss of K in urine, lowered glucose tolerance, uric acid retention (related to hydrochlorothiazide, etc.).

chlorotrianisene: has estrogenic action, with prolonged effect due to storage in fat; is activated after release.

chlorpromazine: phenothiazine; antipsychotic, antiemetic. Side effects include sedation, hypotension, and extrapyramidal actions (e.g., dyskinesias, tremor, rigidity)

cholestyramine: exchange resin; binds bile acids and some drugs (digoxin, thyroxine, anticoagulants) in gut.

cimetidine: histamine H_2-antagonist. Used in treatment of peptic ulcer disease.

cis-platinum: antitumor agent (especially testicular cancer), nephrotoxic.

clindamycin: antibiotic. Side effects include colitis.

clofibrate: lowers blood triglycerides. Used in treatment of hyperlipoproteinemias and for prevention of myocardial infarction. Latter use is controversial.

clonidine: antihypertensive, acting in central nervous system, α-adrenergic. Blood pressure may rebound excessively following sudden withdrawal.

codeine: opioid narcotic analgesic (weak); suppresses cough.

colchicine: plant alkaloid, antimitotic. Used as antiinflammatory drug in acute gout attacks.

corticosteroids: natural and synthetic steroids like those produced by adrenal cortex (adrenocorticosteroids). Hydrocortisone (cortisol), prednisolone, betamethasone, etc. Antiinflammatory agents; used to treat asthma, etc. Wide spectrum of side effects includes Na retention, K loss, hyperglycemia, peptic ulcer, inhibition of growth, osteomalacia, psychosis.

corticotropin: adrenocorticotropin, ACTH, peptide hormone. Found in anterior pituitary. Used in tests of pituitary–adrenal cortex axis function. Used instead of corticosteroids sometimes, especially in children.

crotamine: peptide from rattlesnake venom; increases Na permeability of cell membranes.

cyclophosphamide: cytotoxic drug. Used in cancer chemotherapy (especially Hodgkin's disease and lymphosarcoma). Can be carcinogenic.

cytochalasins: metabolites isolated from molds; can inhibit cell activities by breaking microfilament systems.

cytotoxic drugs: used in cancer chemotherapy.

DDAVP: analogue of ADH, deamino-D-arginine vasopressin. Used in treatment of central diabetes insipidus (= desmopressin). Prolonged action, 10 to 20 hours; low vasopressor effect.

DDT: insecticide.

demeclocycline: antibiotic (tetracycline group); may block action of ADH on kidney.

DES: see *diethylstilbestrol*.

desmopressin: analogue of ADH. Used in treatment of central diabetes insipidus. See *DDAVP*.

DFP: diisofluorophosphate; irreversible inhibitor of cholinesterase. Used in treatment of glaucoma.

diazoxide: hypotensive drug for hypertensive emergencies; hyperglycemic (for insulinoma); relaxes uterus for delaying labor. Side effects include Na retention, tachycardia, hyperglycemia.

dieldrin: insecticide; can be absorbed through skin.

diethylstilbestrol (DES): nonsteroid estrogen. Used in menopausal disorders (may result in uterine cancer), "at-risk" pregnancies (has resulted in adenocarcinoma of vagina and cervix in the children of recipients), cancer of prostate. Additive to animal feed (now mostly discontinued).

digoxin: see *cardiac glycosides*.

L-dopa: used in treatment of parkinsonism. Side effects are gastrointestinal, cardiac arrhythmias, dyskinesias.

ecothiophate: cholinesterase inhibitor (irreversible). Used in treatment of glaucoma; may cause cataracts.

endorphins: natural peptides from brain, with analgesic properties.

epinephrine: natural catecholamine hormone secreted by adrenal medulla; increases blood pressure and blood glucose, relaxes bronchus.

estradiol: estrogen (which see) steroid sex hormone from ovaries.

estrogens: natural steroid hormones from ovaries. Analogues include diethylstilbestrol (DES), ethinylestradiol, mestranol, etc. Used for menopausal disorders, cancer therapy, oral contraceptives, etc.

ethacrynic acid: diuretic drug (potent). Used in treatment of hypertension, congestive heart failure, edema. Side effects include hypokalemia, deafness, hypovolemia.

ethanol: recreational and addictive drug. Used as skin antiseptic, and for delay of labor.

ethisterone: progestin derivative of testosterone. Used in disorders of female reproductive system.

furosemide: diuretic (potent). Used in treatment of hypertension, congestive heart failure, edema. Side effects include hypokalemia, hypovolemia, metabolic alkalosis.

glucagon: peptide hormone from A-cells of islets of Langerhans; has hyperglycemic action. Used in treatment of insulin hypoglycemia.

glutethimide: nonbarbiturate sedative-hypnotic, addictive.

griseofulvin: antifungal drug used in infections of skin, hair, and nails.

growth hormone: protein hormone from anterior pituitary. Used in treatment of pituitary dwarfism.

guanethidine: adrenergic blocker; depletes stores of norepinephrine in peripheral nerves. Used in treatment of moderate to severe hypertension. Side effects include postural hypotension, fluid retention.

halothane: general anesthetic; relaxes smooth muscle (vascular and uterine); possibly is hepatotoxic.

hexamethonium: ganglionic blocker; once had limited use as antihypertensive drug. Disadvantages: must be frequently injected and has wide range of side effects due to blockade of both parasympathetic and sympathetic nerves.

hexobarbital: barbiturate. Used intravenously for general anesthesia (short-acting).

hydralazine: hypotensive; has direct action on vascular muscle. Used in treatment of hypertension. Side effects include tachycardia (reflex), lupus erythematosus–like syndrome at higher doses.

hydrocortisone sodium succinate: corticosteroid for intravenous use in emergencies (e.g., status asthmaticus, Addisonian crisis).

imipramine: tricyclic antidepressant used in affective disorders. Side effects often reflect anticholinergic action.

indomethacin: antiinflammatory. Side effects are common, including effects on gut and CNS (headache, dizziness confusion). Aplastic anemia can occur.

insulin: natural peptide hormone from B-cells of islets of Langerhans. Used in treatment of diabetes mellitus. Current sources mainly pigs and cattle, but human insulin (from cloned bacteria) may become available soon.

isoniazid: antibacterial. Used in treatment of tuberculosis. Side effects not common but can reflect action on nervous system (CNS and peripheral).

isoproterenol: beta-adrenergic agonist drug once used as bronchodilator, as in asthma. Side effects are related to action on heart; tachycardia, arrythmias.

lithium: used in treatment of manic depression. Side effects include tremor and slurred speech. Can inhibit action of ADH and release of thyroid hormones.

local anesthetics: procaine, lidocaine etc. Used for anesthesia at local sites; in dentistry, eye, etc.

lysine vasopressin: natural analogue (in pigs) of ADH. Used in treatment of diabetes insipidus.

mefenamic acid: antiinflammatory drug. High incidence of side effects, including actions on CNS and agranulocytosis, limits its use.

meprobamate: tranquilizer. Addiction can occur.

methotrexate: cytotoxic drug, antimetabolite. Used in cancer therapy.

α-methyldopa: antihypertensive drug (adrenergic block), with site of action mainly in CNS. Side effects include sedation, reversible liver damage, and, rarely, hemolytic anemia.

methyltestosterone: analogue male sex hormone, with androgenic-anabolic activity. Used in treatment of hypogonadal conditions. Hepatotoxic.

metyrapone: inhibits adrenal cortex. Used in treatment of hyperadrenocortisolism and in tests of adrenocortical function.

mineral oil (paraffin oil): laxative; now obsolete. Can interfere with absorption of fat-soluble nutrients.

mitotane: inhibits adrenal cortex. Used in treatment of adrenal cancer.

monensin: carboxylic acid, Na ionophore (not used therapeutically).

monoamine oxidase inhibitors: antidepressant drugs (e.g., phenelzine, tranylcypromine, nialamide). Can interact with tyramine in food to produce hypertensive crisis.

morphine: opioid narcotic analgesic, drug of addiction.

nalidixic acid: antibacterial drug. Used principally for urinary tract infections.

nalorphine: opioid antagonist. Some agonist activity remains, so not preferred for treatment of opioid intoxication.

naloxone: opioid antagonist. Used in treatment of overdose of opioid drugs.

neomycin: wide-spectrum antibiotic. Mostly used topically for infections of integument.

nialamide: monoamine oxidase inhibitor (which see). Used to treat psychiatric disorders.

nicotine: ingredient of tobacco. Used for stimulation of CNS.

nigericin: carboxylic acid, K ionophore (not used therapeutically).

nitroprusside (Na salt): potent hypotensive drug. Used intravenously in hypertensive emergencies.

norepinephrine: adrenergic neurotransmitter.

norethindrone: progestin, derivative of testosterone. Used in oral contraceptives and disorders of female reproductive system.

nortriptylene: tricyclic antidepressant. Used in affective disorders.

opium: mixture of opioid compounds from poppy (*Papaver somniferum*); addictive. Still used sometimes for treatment of diarrhea and for analgesia.

oral contraceptives ("the Pill"): usually mixtures of progestins and estrogens that prevent conception. Serious (but rare) side effects include thromboembolic and cardiovascular disorders.

oxyphenbutazone: antiinflammatory drug. High incidence of side effects occurs, including peptic ulceration and agranulocytosis.

oxytocin: natural peptide hormone of neurohypophysis. Used in induction of labor; prevents postpartum hemorrhage.

penicillin: antibiotic, originally from *Penicillium* mold, now a family of different compounds (e.g., penicillin G, oxacillin, ampicillin). Serious hypersensitivity reactions can occur.

pentazocine: weak analgesic on which some physical dependence develops. Side effects are not uncommon at higher doses (sedation, sweating, dizziness, nausea, etc.).

perchlorate: antithyroid agent used for test of thyroid function. Possibility of aplastic anemia excludes chronic use.

pethidine (meperidine): narcotic analgesic, addictive, with shorter duration of action than morphine (one-tenth as potent). Has atropine-like side effects. Sometimes used in labor, but crosses placenta.

phenacetin: nonnarcotic antipyretic analgesic, usually dispensed in mixtures of such drugs. Implicated in genesis of analgesic nephropathy (necrosis of renal papilla); use restricted.

phenformin: biguanide oral hypoglycemic (antidiabetic drug). Used in treatment of mature-onset diabetes mellitus. Withdrawn in United States, as can precipitate lactic acidosis.

phenobarbital: sedative, hypnotic, anticonvulsant drug; addictive.

phenolphthalein: laxative.

phenothiazines: antipsychotic drugs, antiemetics (e.g., chlorpromazine, prochlorperazine). Some physical dependence may occur. Side effects include postural hypotension and extrapyramidal effects (rigidity, tremor, dyskinesia).

phenoxybenzamine: α-adrenergic antagonist. Used in treatment of pheochromocytoma (excess epinephrine and norepinephrine from adrenal medullary tumors).

phenylbutazone: has antiinflammatory action. See *oxyphenbutazone* for side effects.

phenytoin (diphenylhydantoin): anticonvulsant drug. Used for treatment of epilepsy, also as antiarrhythmic (heart). Hyperplasia of gums common; hypersensitivity (allergic) reactions may develop.

prazosin: antihypertensive drug, with direct action on peripheral vascular muscle. May initially result in fainting due to sudden hypotensive action.

primaquine: antimalarial drug. May result in hemolysis in genetically predisposed individuals.

primidone: anticonvulsant drug. Used in treatment of epilepsy. Phenobarbital is one of its active metabolites.

probenecid: uricosuric drug. Used in treatment of gout. Originally developed to block penicillin excretion in urine.

procainamide: antiarrhythmic (heart) drug, especially of ventricle. Lupus erythematosus-like syndrome may develop.

progesterone: natural steroid hormone from ovaries.

prontosil: prototype sulfonamide antimicrobial drug.

propoxyphene (Darvon): analgesic; may be habit-forming. Effectiveness as analgesic in doubt.

propranolol: β-adrenergic antagonist. Used in treatment of hypertension, angina, and cardiac arrhythmias. Can result in bronchospasm in asthmatics or heart failure in predisposed individuals. Contraindicated in diabetes mellitus.

propylthiouracil: antithyroid drug. Agranulocytosis may occur (rarely).

prostaglandins: natural fatty acids. Ubiquitous distribution and effects. Used for induction of labor and abortions.

puromycin: antibiotic; inhibits cell protein formation, translation on ribosomes. Used in chemotherapy of trypanosome infections.

quinidine: cardiac antiarrhythmic drug, especially atrial fibrillation. Side effects include cinchonism (deafness), hypersensitivity reactions.

quinine: antimalarial drug. Side effects include cinchonism (deafness) and hypersensitivity reactions.

reserpine: antihypertensive; adrenergic blocking agent. Depletes stores of norepinephrine in nerve endings. Side effects include psychosis and peptic ulcer.

salbutamol: β$_2$-adrenergic agonist. Used in treatment of asthma and emphysema.

salicylates: analgesic, antiinflammatory, antipyretic drugs. Sodium salicylate, aspirin.

spironolactone: potassium-sparing diuretic, aldosterone antagonist. Side effects include hyperkalemia, gynecomastia, menstrual disorders.

streptomycin: aminoglycoside antibiotic. Side effects include deafness, neuromuscular blockade, and hypersensitivity reactions.

succinylcholine: neuromuscular blocking drug (depolarizing type). Used as muscle relaxant in anesthesia.

sulfacetamide: sulfonamide antibacterial. Used for ophthalmic infections.

sulfaphenazole: sulfonamide antibacterial.

sulfonamides: antimicrobial drugs. Generic name for derivatives of sulfanilamide.

sulfonylureas: oral hypoglycemic antidiabetic drugs; tolbutamide, acetohexamide, tolazamide, chlorpropamide, glibenclamide. Used for treatment of mature-onset diabetes mellitus.

tamoxifen: antiestrogen. Used in treatment of breast cancer.

tetracycline: antibiotic with wide spectrum of actions and side effects.

tetrodotoxin: paralytic poison from puffer fish, etc.; blocks Na-channels in nerve and muscle.

thalidomide: nonbarbiturate sedative. Resulted in birth defects; no longer used.

theophylline: xanthine alkaloid; relaxes bronchus in asthma, provides cardiac stimulation in acute congestive heart failure.

thiazides: diuretics; chlorothiazide (which see), hydrochlorothiazide, etc.

thiocyanate: has antithyroid and hypotensive activity. Widespread side effects exclude therapeutic use.

thiopental: barbiturate, fast-acting. Used intravenously as general anesthetic.

thiouracils: antithyroid drugs. See *propylthiouracil*.

thromboxanes: active metabolites of prostaglandins.

thyroxine (T_4): natural hormone of thyroid gland. Used for hormone replacement. Illicit use for weight reduction. Overdose can result in dangerous cardiac arrhythmias.

ticrynafen: uricosuric diuretic. Withdrawn owing to incidence of hepatic and kidney disorders.

triampterine: potassium-sparing diuretic, with weak diuretic effect. Used in conjunction with other diuretics to compensate for K loss.

triiodothyronine (T_3): natural hormone of thyroid gland. Used for hormone replacement. Can result in cardiac arrhythmias.

tubocurarine: neuromuscular blocking drug (nondepolarizing type). Used as muscle relaxant in anesthesia.

valinomycin: peptide, K ionophore (not used therapeutically).

vasopressin: peptide, antidiuretic hormone (ADH). Used in treatment of diabetes insipidus.

veratridine: plant alkaloid; lowers blood pressure and induces vomiting.

vincristine: cytotoxic (antimetabolite) drug. Used in treatment of cancers, Hodgkin's disease, and lymphomas.

vitamin D_3: dihydrocholecalciferol, natural prohormone. Used in treatment of disorders of calcium metabolism.

Index

absorption of drugs, 13, 34, 102, 118
abstinence syndrome, 95
acetylation of drugs, 25, 91
addiction, 96
adenylate cyclase, 60, 87, 99, 100
administration of drugs, 12, 16
adrenergic receptors, 70
adverse effects of drugs, 108
  due to genetic differences, 90
  interactions, 99, 126
  monitoring, 123
  nature of, 111
affinity, 46
agranulocytosis, 116
allergic reactions, 111
Ames test, 117
anaphylactic reactions, 116
antagonists, 49
  competitive, 49
  noncompetitive, 51
antidiuretic hormone, 74

bile, 32
binding of drugs, 19, 21, 29
binding proteins, 19, 21, 29
bioassay, 10
bioavailability of drugs, 9, 16

calcium, 88
carcinogenesis, 116, 131
cardiac, glycosides, 4, 87
cell membrane, 79
"coated pits," 64
cross-tolerance, 94
cytochrome P-450 system, 26

DES (diethylstilbestrol), 122, 129
desensitization, 70
development of new drugs, 129
"disintegration" test, 8
displacement of drugs, from binding, 19

dissociation constant, K_D, 59
dissolution test, 8
dissolution time, 18
distribution of drugs, 18
dose–response curves, 45
"down regulation," 68
drug abuse, 96
drug dependence, 94, 96, 97
drug interactions, 31, 99, 126
drug–receptor interactions, 53
drug resistance, 94
drug trials, 130
duration of action of drugs, 14

ED_{50}, 89
ED50, 45, 47
efficacy, 46
elimination rate constant, k_e, 35, 38
endorphins, 98
enterohepatic circulation, 33
environmental chemicals, 126
equilibrium association constant, K_a, 46
equilibrium dissociation constant, K_D, 46, 59
excretion of drugs, 20, 32, 103

Ferguson principle, 41
folic acid antagonists, 121
food–drug interactions, 128
fractional absorption, f, 38

generic drugs, 7
glucuronidation of drugs, 27, 32
goiter, 127

habituation, 95
half-life, for elimination, $t_{1/2}$, 35, 38
hemolysis, 116
hemolytic anemia, 116

induction of enzymes, 30, 118

infants, 29, 33, 119, 131
insulin, 56, 58, 68
insulin receptor, 68
intrinsic activity, 46
ionization of drugs, 82
ionophores, 86

$K_{D\ activation}$, 59
$K_{D\ apparent}$, 59
$K_{D\ binding}$, 59
kidney and drug excretion, 20, 32, 111
kidney disease, and drug clearance, 29, 111

LD_{50}, 89
lethal dose, 89, 131
lipid solubility, 80
liver and drug metabolism, 22, 30, 118
liver disease, and drug clearance, 29, 111

mechanisms of action, of drugs, 40
MEDISC, 124
metabolism of drugs, 22, 103, 130
mobile receptor theory, 63, 65
morphine, 67, 96
multiple doses of drugs, 35, 37

negative cooperativity, 66, 68, 71
nuclear receptors, 62, 63

occupation theory, 44
opiate receptors, 67, 98
opiates, 96
oral contraceptives, 127
oxidative metabolism of drug, 25
oxytocin, 74

pA_2, 52
partial agonists, 51
partition coefficient, 80
penicillin, 4, 33
pharmacodynamics, 2, 102
pharmacogenetics, 2, 90
pharmacokinetics, 2, 33, 102
pK_a, 82
plasma membrane, 79
potency, 47
primaquine sensitivity, 92

prolongation of action of drugs, 14
proprietary drugs, 7
psychogenic dependence, 95
pumps for drug administration, 15

QSAR, 72

"rapid inactivators," 91
rate theory, 52
receptor reserve, 51
receptors, 41, 42, 61
    architecture of, 64
    control of, 69
    identification, 55
    interaction with drugs, 53
    nature of, 61
    number of, 61, 69
    structure, 64
receptor theory, 44
reduction metabolism of drugs, 27
responses to drugs, 40

Scatchard plots, 57, 60
serum sickness, 116
side effects, 106, 123
"slow inactivators," 91
sodium-channels, 84
sodium-potassium activated ATPase, 86
sources of drugs, 7, 129
spare receptors, 51
speed of onset of drugs, 14
steroid hormone receptors, 62, 63
structure–activity relationships (SAR), 30, 72

tachyphylaxis, 93
teratogenesis, 119, 131, 132
tertiary structure of drugs, 53, 73
thalidomide, 122, 132
therapeutic index, 89
thrombocytopenia, 116
tobacco, 127
tolerance, 93, 94
toxic effects of drugs, 106, 123, 131

vehicles for drugs, 15
volume of distribution, V_d, 35, 38

withdrawal illness, 95